TANTRIC SECRETS

FOR MEN

TANTRIC SECRETS

FOR MEN

What Every Woman Will Want Her Man to Know about Enhancing Sexual Ecstasy

Kerry Riley with Diane Riley

Destiny Books

Rochester, Vermont

Destiny Books
One Park Street
Rochester, Vermont 05767
www.InnerTraditions.com

Destiny Books is a division of Inner Traditions International

*Note to the reader: The purpose of this book is to educate and inform. The authors are not
engaged in rendering medical or psychological services. If medical or other expert assistance
is required the services of a competent professional should be sought. The authors and publisher
disclaim any responsiblilty or liability for individuals who engage in any of the sexual
practices described in this book.*

LIBRARY OF CONGRESS CATALOGING-IN-PUBLICATION DATA
Riley, Kerry.
Tantric secrets for men : what every woman will want her man to know
about enhancing sexual ecstasy / Kerry Riley with Diane Riley.
p. cm.
ISBN 0-89281-969-3
1. Sex instruction for men. 2. Tantrism. I. Riley, Diane. II. Title.

HQ36 .R528 2002
613.9'6—dc21
2002013451

Printed and bound in the United States

10   9   8   7   6   5   4   3   2   1

Text design and layout by Peri Champine
This book was typeset in Bembo with Bodega Sans as the display typeface

Contents

Acknowledgments

I thank my partner in life, my wife, Diane, for sharing this journey into love with me. I thank her for expanding my understanding of the divine feminine, of what's important to women, and for all the love, joy, and sexual passion we have together. She has been my greatest teacher.

My grateful appreciation goes to all the teachers on our path, especially Larry Collins, Dr. Stephen Chang, David and Ellen Ramsdale, Charles and Caroline Muir, Marty and Ruth and teachers of More University, Elliot and Hollie Tanza, Betty Bethards, Neville Rowe, Bill Spence, and De Raj.

I also wish to thank all those whose books or workshops have helped us, especially Osho Rajneesh and Neslish and Satyo for their heart-opening work. And those who assisted me at the beginning of my personal development work—Daniel and Marcea Webber, John Kehoe, Martyn Jackson, Dr. Masahiro Oki, Masunaga Sensai, and Satyananda teachers.

Special thanks to the many students who have attended the seminars Diane and I conduct. Your examples continue to inspire me to teach these secrets from the heart, knowing absolutely that they work for anyone who applies them. Thank you for your positive feedback and for sharing your stories. Special thanks to Tim and to Nola, for her assistance with the editing of the book, and to my agent, Ellen Ramsdale, for her invaluable work in securing our publisher.

I am grateful also to my mother, father, and brother for all the unconditional love I've had. And finally blessings to our children, Soelae, Lisa, and Sam, for continually connecting me with my heart and reminding me of the value of love in my life.

Preface

Imagine having a partner who says that she couldn't possibly have a better lover than you, that she can't wait for you to come home each day. Imagine being in a relationship that is exciting, sexy, and emotionally nurturing; being able to make love as long as you want, as many times as you like, at any age, and knowing absolutely that you can satisfy your partner, not just physically but on every level of being—body, heart, and soul.

Imagine continuing to explore and create together fulfilling and profound lovemaking experiences; continuing to grow and bond with greater intimacy, loving feelings, and communication. Imagine feeling more pleasure, with deeper, stronger orgasms, for you and your partner.

Lovemaking that will bring more love, joy, and pleasure into your life is possible.

Held within these pages are secrets and practices that will turn this dream into reality, secrets you will treasure for a lifetime. The secrets I share in this book are not theoretical—they are practices that my wife, Diane, and I have developed through actual experience of working successfully with thousands of people over many years. I am not suggesting that by reading this book you'll never have another problem in your relationship. Diane and I have been married for more than twenty years and we have three children: I know that difficulties will continue to arise! Yet I've also invested many years of my life finding out what it takes to sustain love and sexual passion with the same woman. The old proverb "Blessed is the man who has found his work and one woman to love" rings as true in our lifetimes as it ever has.

This book is for any man of any age who desires to be an extraordinary lover. Any man who knows he can satisfy a woman feels ten feet tall. Much of a man's self-image is tied up with how good he feels he is as a lover. Every man wants to be good in bed. For my father's generation that was relatively easy: you just moved in and out until you felt an explosion of energy. That's all there was to it. The only challenge was in finding a willing partner.

In the 1960s, my older brother's era, everything changed. Men began to realize that their pleasure in sex was magnified when their partner was also experiencing a great amount of pleasure. Men realized that in order to be good lovers they needed to warm up their partner with lots of foreplay. While men were suddenly challenged to bring women to orgasm, there wasn't a lot of pressure to succeed because, throughout the previous two thousand years, women's sexuality had been suppressed. It was common for women to be uncomfortable with their sexuality and to have difficulty reaching orgasm. If orgasm happened, that was great, but if it didn't, it wasn't such a big deal because it was accepted that "good girls don't do it anyway." Lovemaking continued to be mostly about the man's pleasure.

Today, being a good lover is more challenging than it has ever been. Women are on the other side of a sexual revolution. Women today don't simply want sex; they want great sex, which includes emotional as well as physical nourishment. Many men go into lovemaking concerned that they won't be able to meet their partners' needs.

I would suggest that what we must do as self-aware men is work with our partners as teammates in continuing to support and nourish this opening of women's sexuality. One of the best ways we can do this is by becoming extraordinary lovers. The message of *Tantric Secrets for Men* is powerful and yet simple—truly great sex is much more than just physical contact; it combines sexual pleasure with love and deep intimacy. This book will show you how you can reach heightened states of ecstasy and pleasure together. It contains information that can make any man not just a good lover, but a truly extraordinary and caring lover. And the truth is, that is what every woman yearns for in a man.

So often in lovemaking a woman doesn't ask for what she wants, either because she's not sure of what she wants or she's afraid she will hurt her partner's feelings. Often the man doesn't ask because he's "supposed to" know. And we wonder why sexual loving loses its original spark after several years, or even months, with the same partner! Sexual love is the fuel for a passionate relationship. Without this it's like having a car without gas: you have the car but the engine doesn't spark and you can't go anywhere. We can all do with some new fuel in our love lives.

I believe that there is a "new man" in the world today, one who wants to experience sex at its full potential, who desires to make love in such a way that it opens the door to the greatest joy for his loved one and himself and fulfills his deepest yearnings. This new, aware man realizes the importance of learning about love, sex, and relationship. He is strongly conscious of the centrality of these matters in his life, and he wants to learn all there is about lovemaking. Yet there is very little good education available on how to become a good lover. And contrary to what the ego would have us men believe, we are not born naturally great at lovemaking.

I am not talking about intercourse here; anyone can do that. I'm talking about learning how to make love so that you can nourish a woman on every level of her being—body, heart, and soul. I am speaking about making love in such a way that your woman not only experiences levels of physical pleasure beyond anything she has ever known before, but also feels a deep love in her heart and experiences an ecstasy that transcends her sense of time, space, and thought.

The secrets in this book will give you the knowledge and skills to be an extraordinary lover for your partner. Every woman wants her man to know these secrets. Once you know how to nourish a woman on this level your relationship will reach new depths of love and new heights of ecstasy. The benefits of knowing these secrets are not only that you nourish your partner's sexuality better than any other man can, but that you learn how to access higher states of pleasure yourself.

Most men have neglected exploring many aspects of their sexuality with their loved one. In recent years the general focus in sexual relations has been so much on giving women an orgasm that the man's pleasure is often determined by the woman's orgasmic response. A lot of men don't realize this until they learn the secrets of sexual fulfillment and begin to explore, with their partner, higher orgasmic states for themselves. The secrets revealed here are not only about physical pleasure. They will also show you how to open up and feel the love that is in your heart much more deeply while you are making love. Once your partner experiences this heartfelt love she will be more open to making love, she will want to make love more often, and there will be more sexual energy available for both of you.

Very early in my studies I learned a great sexual secret—that it is better to give a woman a little of what she truly wants than a lot of what you think she wants!

By the end of this book you are going to know more about lovemaking than 98 percent of men on the planet, and the woman you have in your life (or the one you attract to you) will love you for it because you will bring to her the love and pleasure she has always dreamed of. In response, her love and sexual energy toward you will know no bounds!

Some men will think "I already know all there is to know. I have tried all the positions, I know about the clitoris and the G-spot, and I practice oral sex. What more is there?" This attitude is understandable because there has been very little quality education about sexual loving available in our society. *Tantric Secrets for Men* is about to change that. This book not only explains techniques, it asks you some key questions, such as: Have you explored how much love you can feel while making love? Have you explored going into heightened states of ecstasy, not just during climax but for fifteen-minute periods? Have you experienced using your lovemaking as a devotion, as a spiritual experience? In *Tantric Secrets for Men* I outline:

- How to reach heightened states of ecstasy and pleasure beyond realms you have explored so far.
- How to open to love in such a way that your heart opens for your partner and you remember how great it feels to be deeply, passionately "in love."
- How to transform your lovemaking into a sacred experience that touches you and your woman on every level of your being.
- How to create and sustain a fulfilling relationship in which you keep the magic of love alive.

In the workshops Diane and I conduct I often ask the men: "What do you imagine you will be thinking about at the end of your life?" I guarantee that on your deathbed you won't be thinking about your best day at the office! You will reflect on who you loved and how much love you allowed into your life—including your sexual loving, one of the most intimate interactions you can have with another human being.

No matter what your age, you are about to go on an adventure, a new journey into sexual loving. There is enough fuel in this book to keep you and your partner charged and in love throughout your lives. Enjoy!

Note: In *Tantric Secrets for Men* I am addressing heterosexual men and women because this is where my experience lies. However, the same principles can be adapted to suit your preference in sexual relationships; many gay couples tell us they benefit immensely from our tantra courses. They will benefit from this book as well.

1

Lovemaking as a Spiritual Experience

It is written in the ancient texts of China and India that it was common for emperors, kings, and noblemen trained in the art of lovemaking to be passionate lovers in their nineties with up to twenty consorts, all of whom they were keeping sexually satisfied. In the ruling class a man's power was measured by the number of consorts he could keep satisfied. A husband was respected more for keeping his wife sexually satisfied than for anything else. In the ancient cultures of Egypt, Arabia, India, Nepal, Tibet, China, and Japan polygamy was common, so it was essential for a man to know the arts of lovemaking.

In Chinese Taoist texts it is written that the emperor should make love to nine chosen consorts every night, progressing from the lower ranks to the higher. In their book *Sexual Secrets: The Alchemy of Ecstasy*, authors Nik Douglas and Penny Slinger quote from an ancient Chinese text: "Retaining his semen by proficiency in the Art of Love, the Emperor concentrates powers within. Then, at the full moon, he bestows his seed on the Queen of Heaven." A child born from such a ritual was purported to have magical powers.

Most men these days ejaculate within the first fifteen minutes of being engaged in lovemaking; they wouldn't have commanded much respect in ancient China. Our education and proficiency in the art of lovemaking is lacking in our modern day, yet every man has the ability to master these sexual skills.

One of the reasons I was attracted to these studies of eroticism and ecstasy is because ancient texts from the East teach that sex was sacred. I like the idea of my lovemaking being sacred. I don't use the term *sacred* here in the conventional religious sense of something existing above us somewhere. Such a view tends to split reality into two parts, with a degraded Earth below and a pure holy Heaven on high. Things on this earthly plane can be sacred if we have the eyes to see the sacredness in them: the sacred order of Earth and sky, of life and death, of the mind and the heart and the body.

We can view human existence itself as sacred, and, if we choose, we can see lovemaking as sacred.

Many people today are seeking spiritual growth. When I tell them that Diane and I use our sexual love as a way of becoming more spiritual they are quite shocked. This probably stems from the fact that many religions proclaim that if we want to become spiritual we must deny our earthly pleasures. Traditionally in Eastern and Western cultures, celibacy was a requirement for those who sought a spiritual life.

As a child I was taught, as I'm sure many people were, that the way to God was through prayer and going to church. However, these things never really gave me any profound experience of God. In the mid-1970s I traveled through India where I was introduced to meditation as a practice for spiritual growth. When I practiced meditation it did give me an experience that I felt was spiritual. In the East this was called a mystical experience.

A mystical, or spiritual, experience is foreign to most westerners. A mystical state is not easy to describe, and yet anyone who has had the experience recognizes it. People describe certain common elements in mystical experiences, such as a sense of tranquillity, of timelessness, of intense awareness that everything you see is vivid and everything you touch is very alive; a transcendence from the thoughts of daily life; an expansion of consciousness; a feeling of being connected with the cosmos or at unity with all things. Some say they have a tangible experience of God; others experience the bliss of union with the Divine.

Some of these elements can be present during lovemaking, and when they are it is important to acknowledge this as a spiritual experience. Being in a heightened orgasmic state is a mystical experience. Ancient spiritual systems such as Taoism and tantra readily acknowledge this.

TANTRA AND TAOISM

Tantra, a spiritual science from ancient India, and Taoism, from ancient China, are similar in their basic essence. Both involve balancing the male and female energies to create harmony, and both have an ultimate goal of spiritual unity with the universe or the source or the God within.

The tantric interplay of the male and female energies was represented in Hindu mythology by Shakti and Shiva, and in Taoism by yin and yang. Both tantra and Taoism aim to create union of body, mind, and spirit. In both traditions sexuality is seen and practiced in a spiritual context.

One of the differences between tantra and Taoism is that tantra is filled with rituals and religious deities, gods and goddesses, whereas Taoism is more scientific in its approach. People who are more intuitive or "right-brain" oriented would likely be more attracted to tantra, while those who are more rational and logical, more "left-brain" oriented, would likely be attracted to Taoism, although this is certainly not a rule.

In the seminars that Diane and I conduct we find that women are generally more attracted to the tantric approach and men more to the Taoist approach, at least initially. However, as men open their heart centers more and become deeply connected with their women, they move forward into the tantric approach to sexuality.

It is said that tantra is the oldest single source of knowledge concerning the energies of the mind, body, and spirit. It is the origin and essence of yoga, martial arts, t'ai chi, and the grand philosophies of the Buddha, Confucius, and Lao-tzu.

The word *tantra* means "to expand, to be free, to be liberated." If we are to be really free our sexuality should not be repressed; it should be lived in its totality with joy and without guilt. The more we suppress our sexual desires, the more we will be bound by those desires; the more our sexuality is repressed, the more it wants to burst out. The sad thing is that repressed sexuality often bursts out in harmful ways. The evidence of child sexual abuse that has come to light over the past few decades is an example of what can happen as a result of suppression.

Tantra always emphasizes the sacredness in sex; it teaches that there should be no repression or guilt attached to sex. It also teaches that when a man approaches his beloved he should carry a feeling of the sacred, as if he were stepping in to a temple. Tantra claims that, to know the truth about love, you need to accept the sacredness of sex.

Relics of tantric rituals date back nearly five thousand years; tantric texts began to appear within a few centuries of the beginning of the Christian era. It is speculated that Indian tantra, which spread to Tibet, may have originated with ancient Taoists in China, then reentered China hundreds of years later and revitalized Taoist sexual practices. Through the centuries many mainstream religions have frowned on tantra and Taoism because both systems use sexual union as a vehicle to enlightenment, as a way of experiencing a deep connection with God or the cosmos or the Divine or the source of all existence, whatever you call it according to your beliefs. Yet most religious systems make sex taboo, claiming it leads people away from God. This predominant religious approach eventually forced tantric practices underground, where tantric rituals have been kept secret for hundreds of years.

Only recently have tantric and Taoist practices been interpreted, published, and made available for Western study. This has been refreshing and enlightening for many of us because it has helped us to look at love and sex from a different perspective. We start to question our own attitudes and realize how deeply our consciousness has been conditioned by our Christian upbringing, which suggests that sexuality is somehow evil.

We are taught at school that the first sin in the Garden of Eden was committed by Eve when she offered Adam the apple from the Tree of

Life. But that's not a sin. What is sinful is that some sexually insecure man invented a God who couldn't rejoice in Adam and Eve's sexual nature. It's a tremendous mistake that the very act on which the procreation of life depends is depicted as a sin. We have been taught that we must be either spiritual or sexual, that we must not be "drawn to the devil" by bodily pleasures. Even though these days most people would see this teaching as ridiculous, it still subconsciously affects our attitudes toward sex, and we carry this negative conditioning into our lovemaking.

If we were brought up in a culture that revered sexuality it would be much easier to have a healthy attitude toward sex. A tantric attitude toward sex is that sex is God's greatest gift; that it is sacred; that to have pleasure from sex is a prayer to God, a way of showing gratitude for our existence. Tantra sees sexual union as a way of generating lifeforce through the body that is healing, rejuvenating, energizing; it can be used as a meditation to reach mystical states of love and consciousness.

Because tantra covers the full spectrum of life it accepts and reveres sexual love and pleasure. It does not accept any kind of religious, cultural, or tribal inhibitions. It's about exploring the extraordinary in your love and your sexuality, with the only proviso being that it causes the other person or yourself no harm. Tantra teaches that we deserve all the love and sexual pleasure we can possibly receive; that sexual loving is a way to reach the mysteries of the heart, the soul, the god and goddess within each person. It also teaches that sex is a way of bonding with a lover—physically, emotionally, and spiritually—to create feelings of ecstatic pleasure, deep intimacy, and expanded consciousness. It's a way of transcending daily life and the ego to become one with your beloved, to become one with all things, and to invite a tangible experience of God.

Taoists would say that lovemaking is the way to longevity and that by applying certain techniques we can rejuvenate ourselves and awaken our intuitive centers. They also believe that we can use our lovemaking to heal ourselves and our partners, because when we are in heightened states of sexual energy our whole body is charged and the immune system strengthened.

SACRED SEX:
THE DOOR TO ENLIGHTENMENT

Imagine how much more we could embrace our sexuality if we were introduced to such beliefs as tantra and Taoism when we first asked questions about sex. It's important to recognize that any judgments we have about sex reflect our inhibitions and demonstrate that we are not entirely free and accepting of our own sexuality.

What we need is a new ideal for manhood, a man who can take sex back to its original sacredness, who is able to make love in such a way that it opens the door to enlightenment for his beloved and himself and fulfills his deepest yearnings for the meaning of life. We need education in lovemaking because it will increase our choices and our knowledge. We don't have to assume the attitudes handed down to us by society. We can adopt new attitudes that serve us better and help us have a more fulfilling, happy, healthy love life.

Some aspects of tantra and Taoism may seem a little strange at first, especially the link between sexuality and spirituality, but like anything in life we need to consider all approaches and then select what serves us. Of course, sometimes when a new attitude is presented to us we take it on immediately because it rings true for us. At other times we have to let it sit for a while; we put it on the shelf and perhaps use it in years to come. It's important to experiment, to play with innocence and openness as a child plays with a new toy. Parents terrorize their children out of the delight of their sexual experimentation. But we are not children anymore. It's time to choose new ways of exploring sex and love on physical, emotional, and spiritual levels.

A HEALTHY ATTITUDE TOWARD SEX

Having a healthy attitude toward lovemaking makes all the difference to the experience. You can be in exactly the same lovemaking position as someone else, but ultimately it's the mind that creates the experience. If the mind is saying, "I wish this would end," you may have some sort of resistance to pleasure from past conditioning. How could the most sensitive part of the body, with the most nerve endings, not give you pleasure? Have you ever thought about that? If you believe that to make love to reach high states of sexual pleasure is healing, then the experience will be totally different. Our experience of lovemaking is affected by our attitudes. A man who has been conditioned to believe that lovemaking is a spiritual encounter will have a totally different experience from a man who sees it as an opportunity to put another notch in his belt.

Anything that happens in our lovemaking is interpreted first through our attitudes and beliefs. From these we derive our experience. One way to alter our experience is to change our attitudes and beliefs. Some people watching a high tantric experience might see it merely as two people having good sex. So what is the difference between tantra and just having great sex? One of the key differences is where the mind is focused at the moment. It's the same in life. One's experience of life depends on where the mind is. We are all living in the same world, but our differing experiences are determined by our perceptions.

In lovemaking it's not what we are doing that affects us; it's the attitude with which we are doing it that makes the real difference to our experience. If we can internalize the attitude that our lovemaking is spiritual, then our lovemaking will indeed become a spiritual experience.

WAYS TO USE YOUR LOVEMAKING AS A SPIRITUAL PRACTICE

It is valuable to set aside special times to treat your lovemaking as a spiritual practice. Meditation, prayer, ritual, and ceremony are common practices people use on a spiritual path. These can be combined in lovemaking by:

- Creating the right attitude. Say to your partner: "Let's make love as a meditation today." This creates the mind-set that everything you do in this particular session is for your spiritual growth.

- Creating a special space by placing ritual objects on a small table nearby—flowers, incense, candles, and other objects of spiritual significance for you.
- Sitting opposite each other and making a devotion. This is like a prayer in which you can say things such as "May the good energy created by our lovemaking today be devoted to our bonding even closer together," or "May this energy go to the healing of my partner."
- Having a common greeting that you say to each other each time you make love as a spiritual practice. Here is one that Diane and I made up and that we teach to couples. You are welcome to use it if you wish or to make up one that means something special to you. "I honor the Shakti and Shiva within you. I honor your love, your joy, and your pleasure. May our lovemaking today shine light on all things and may the angels of love be with us now." We then ring a special ceremonial bell to send our devotion out to the cosmos.

In this devotion Shakti represents the divine feminine energy within Diane and Shiva represents the divine masculine energy within me. In Hindu mythology it is written that through sexual union we can unite these two forces of the universe, Shakti and Shiva, and have a tangible experience of the Divine. One prevailing Hindu belief is that if you expressed the divinity within your loving union then you would manifest divinity in all aspects of your life. Another Hindu belief is that men and women are channels for God and Goddess. The way for a man to evoke this for himself is to treat his beloved as a goddess. So before I say, "I honor the Shakti within you," I look at Diane and I see beyond her personality, beyond what she has done or said to me, beyond her looks and her actions. I see the goddess who resides in her. At that moment to me she is Shakti, and I feel blessed to be in her presence. As Diane honors the Shiva within me, I feel like Shiva at that moment.

When I say, "I honor your love, your joy, and your pleasure," I'm affirming to her that her love, her joy, and her pleasure are spiritual qualities. When I say "May our lovemaking shine light on all things," I see the love we generate shining light on each other, our family, and the world. The more we can love, the greater our gift to the cosmos.

When I say "May the angels of love be with us now," I think of the tantric belief that when human beings have a deeply loving sexual experience, the angels of love from the cosmos are attracted to the intensity of their vibration.

Now all of this may sound a little strange, but before I knew anything of the Hindu teachings on sexuality something happened to me that convinced me to follow this path of sexuality and spirituality. It's an experience I'll never forget.

It happened after a weeklong workshop that Diane and I were conducting called "Awakening Another Reality," which worked on opening people up to new dimensions physically, mentally, and emotionally. We'd been away in the bush with no telephones or normal time constraints for one week, and when we returned home we were at a very high level of consciousness. Knowing nothing of tantric or Taoist rituals at this time, Diane and I created a lovemaking session that had all the elements of ceremony. After two hours of lovemaking Diane's whole face changed. I had never seen her look so beautiful. She said to me, "Your eyes are gold." She was seeing something beyond me and it felt so wonderful, beyond this earthly plane. After that there was a period of timelessness and no thought.

We woke up later, stunned by the experience and more deeply in love than ever before. We didn't tell anybody about this experience for many years, until we read about a tantric experience almost exactly the same as our own. To us, this extraordinary experience was a gift and a clear message to seek this path in our lives. We both felt blessed.

Seeing the divinity within each other is not such an outrageous proposition. If you go into your lovemaking session with this mind-set it can create a whole new experience for you and broaden the spectrum of the ways you make love. You can play with the idea of Shiva and Shakti and dress as a god and goddess for these special ritual lovemaking sessions. It can become a lot of fun, and spiritual growth should sometimes be fun.

> Your sexuality is not only a vehicle to explore more love; it is also a vehicle for you to find a spiritual path.

LOVEMAKING AS A MEDITATION

In meditation the mind is given something to focus on—sometimes the breath, sometimes a candle flame, sometimes a mantra (a sound you repeat over and over to yourself). These are all techniques to calm the mind and direct the thoughts away from the details of daily life in order to experience a deep inner peace. Later in the book I will give you several techniques that use the breath and certain muscles and that focus on the energy exchange between you and your partner to help keep the mind present in the moment during lovemaking. Meanwhile, here is a simple technique to start with.

ATTENTION ON THE BREATH

Every time you find your mind drifting off or focusing on performance or becoming goal oriented, take your attention back to your breathing: "I am breathing in. I am breathing out," or try coordinating your breathing with your partner's. Follow her breath so you are breathing as one body.

At first the techniques may seem to be creating the experience, but what is really creating it is your ability to be totally present. Your thoughts and feelings and your experience are all one.

> (≈
> (≈   Sexual ecstasy happens when you are so
> (≈   thoroughly absorbed in the richness of
>   the present moment that nothing else
> (≈   exists.

What happens for most couples when they make love is that there are four "people" present: you and your thoughts and your partner and her thoughts, and those thoughts very often are not on the moment at hand. When you are both focusing on the breath and the energy, both minds are attuned. It is possible to have an experience of being one body, one mind, one breath.

The techniques of breath focus and mind focus are very effective in creating a joint meditative experience. However, many people make the mistake of thinking it's the techniques that are creating these magical experiences, so they learn more and more mental techniques, adding *mantras* (sounds) and *yantras* (visual shapes and colors) and experimenting with all kinds of cycles of energy between each other. Their lovemaking becomes more and more a mind experience in which the whole natural beauty of sexual loving is lost.

My advice is to keep it simple. The techniques in chapter 8 are enough to create a meditative experience. By practicing these techniques many times, eventually they become natural during lovemaking. In advanced stages of meditation you achieve a "no mind" state—no program, no rehearsal, no goal, totally being in the present moment. The more familiar you are with the meditative lovemaking experience the easier it becomes to bring meditation naturally into your everyday lovemaking without constantly thinking about techniques.

If, while making love, you are aware that your mind is focusing on performance and result and not on the present moment, then you have the techniques to get you back into the present moment. Once you are in that moment again, forget the techniques, relax, let the breathing be slow and gentle, and go with the flow of energy that is naturally happening. Don't force anything. Don't be goal oriented; be in the here and now as much as possible. Enjoy the meeting of the two bodies and two souls and melt into each other. If you find the mind drifting again or focusing on the result, gently bring it back with your breath. Then be totally present again, feeling every sensation, every touch, every subtle movement of energy that happens.

In practicing lovemaking as a meditation, you will go through four stages that normally occur when learning something new.

Stage 1: Unconscious incompetence—You are not aware that lovemaking can be a meditative experience and you have no skills to make it so.

Stage 2: Conscious incompetence—You become aware that you are not very good at being present with your lovemaking, that your mind is very often focusing on being able to satisfy your partner or on what you are going to do next or on comparing what's happening now with a past experience and trying to repeat it.

Stage 3: Conscious competence—You are consciously bringing your mind into the present moment. You become very confident with the techniques of keeping your mind present on the energy exchange.

Stage 4: Unconscious competence—It happens naturally and you surrender totally to the flow of energy that is occurring between you. Your breathing is slow, you are relaxed, and you've totally let go. A deep silent communication happens between you; you melt into your beloved; your separateness disappears. You become one body, the lovemaking becomes less sexual and more spiritual, and you remain there for hours.

It's usually much easier for you to have this experience when your partner is on top because then you can relax more and surrender to receiving rather than doing.

A WORD ABOUT LANGUAGE

I have tried to avoid using too many terms from Eastern lovemaking traditions because some people may find them awkward and foreign to use or may think the words have spiritual or religious overtones, as many of these traditions combined sexuality with spirituality.

However, in our seminars, tapes, and videos Diane and I borrow a few terms from tantric writings from ancient India because they suit our approach to lovemaking by adding some romantic language and specialness. For the word *penis* we use *lingam,* which means "wand of light." For *vagina* we use the Indian word *yoni,* which means "sacred place, hidden valley, field of pleasure." Diane says she takes her vagina to see a gynecologist but she brings her yoni, her sacred place, to our lovemaking.

2

Learning to Understand Women and Their Needs

In working with numerous groups of men discussing their relationships with women, I've found that men often have similar difficulties. They all say that their partners often behave in ways they don't understand and that they often don't understand their woman's moods and actions.

One exercise I have done frequently with men participating in my courses is to give them a sheet of paper headed: What I find difficult about a woman is . . . Underneath they list the things that come to mind. You can do this practice yourself. For example, Gary wrote the following:

What I find difficult about a woman is:

- She spends hours getting ready to go out.
- Moods—I don't know what causes them, but she seems to have a lot of different moods.
- Spending large sums of money on jewelry.
- Wanting new clothes or shoes every time we get invited to a wedding.
- When she says "nothing's the matter," but you know some-

thing is wrong and you don't know what you've done.

- When you plan to make love that night, then you have a disagreement over dinner and then it's all off in bed as well, even though she promised you through the day.
- Worrying about her weight all the time or the shape of some part of her body. No matter how many times I tell her I love her breasts, she just never gets it.

Not all of these things will apply to the women with whom you have been in relationships, but some of them might. You have probably wished many times that women could understand the way you think or that you could understand them better. Men and women are essentially very different. They think differently and often they see things differently. Men often say to me: "Sometimes I feel like I'm living with someone from another planet. My partner gets annoyed and I have no idea what I have said or done to upset her."

Recent scientific research has shown that male and female brains operate in very different manners. Women differ from men physically and emotionally, and they see the world differently. Even though this is often a politically sensitive subject and there is much debate as to whether differences are due to biological or cultural conditioning, the fact is that understanding and appreciating the differences between women and men have assisted the hundreds of couples to whom we have introduced this concept. The popularity of John Gray's book *Men Are From Mars, Women Are From Venus* attests to the fact that a lot of men and women don't fully understand each other and find it valuable to learn practical ways of appreciating these differences instead of resisting them.

In *Tantric Secrets for Men* I provide insights that will assist men in understanding some important aspects of their partners' behavior. I am in no way implying that women are hard to understand and men are not. It obviously works both ways. These insights have been of enormous value in keeping my relationships mutually fulfilling, loving, and growing.

The new science of evolutionary psychology gives some excellent insights into understanding male and female behavior. In an excellent book, *The Sex Contract: The Evolution of Human Behaviour,* anthropologist Dr. Helen Fisher points out that whether you have a creationist view of the world or an evolutionist view, all evidence supports the view that life today is a transformation of life from the past, that everything in the present is a rearrangement of things that existed in the beginning.

So what was sex like in the beginning? At primate level the female attracted the male in order for him to copulate with her and, in effect, reproduce the human race. That basic programming is built in to every species. It is one of our basic biological functions.

Today we obviously don't behave like animals or basic primates, because we have been socialized and we have a choice about whether to have children or not. Nevertheless, in our culture, no matter what behavior is socially accepted, biological programming continues to affect our behavior. Whenever a man sees an appealing woman walk by he is attracted. Watch a group of guys working on a building site. As an attractive woman walks past all work stops for a moment. Observe a guy working hard at his computer when a woman he finds attractive walks into the office. Suddenly everything is lost; for a second he cannot think. The sexual impulse deflects his attention and confuses his mind. I am not saying he would necessarily act on his impulse or that he would even want to if he had the opportunity. Maybe he is already committed and he honors his relationship. Nevertheless, this instinct exists.

The sexual impulse may not only be coming from the man but also from the woman, who may exude sexual energy in a subtle way. In the animal kindgom the female definitely sends out a scent of attraction while she is on heat. She attracts the male with her scent; they then mate and not too long after, he leaves. (Some female spiders do not require the male at all after conception so they often eat the male after mating. I'm glad I'm not a spider!) Originally in the human species it wasn't appropriate for the male to leave because it took many years before the offspring could fend for itself. He was needed to assist with protection and food. This is, of course, not necessarily the case today, but we did evolve from this.

Unlike any other female organism on Earth, women are able to make love throughout their reproductive cycle. It's almost as if nature had wished human beings to make love daily. Biologically, the human female is capable of constant sexual arousal. No other species makes love with such frequency. Women send out subtle energy or vibrations that men are drawn toward. It's been called the "scent of a woman"; whatever it is, it's very attractive. Females have a gift of nature to attract a male.

WOMEN ATTRACT BY NATURE

This basic nature is one reason why your partner might get upset when you don't give her enough attention. She might feel that her attractiveness is not being recognized. Understanding this may help you to stop arguing when, for example, your partner spends lots of money on makeup or creams. There is no use arguing that the potions she buys are a waste of good money. She is not interested; she does not hear you. It's as though you are communicating with an alien. Indeed, it has helped me considerably in my relationship to accept that in some ways women *are* aliens. They often have different priorities from men.

If I look at it this way, then my partner's behavior does not always have to make sense to me. It's a great relief because I used to spend a lot of time trying to understand women.

≋ Female behavior does not have to make sense to a man.

For example, some women will want to buy a new outfit and shoes to go with the outfit whenever a special occasion comes up. Some women seem to buy shoes all the time, even when there isn't a special event on the horizon! You may reason: "She's got plenty of clothes, so why can't she just be like me—simply put on her best suit. It doesn't make sense!" Just remember that it's okay because she's an alien and that's what these aliens do!

(Of course, many men spend lots of money on new clothes and at the hairdresser and plenty of time in front of the mirror preening themselves. It's a good thing that men can now openly tap in to both their feminine and masculine sides without inhibition. However, when a man starts to become preoccupied with his own attractiveness and gives more attention to that than to noticing and acknowledging his partner's attractiveness, he is heading for trouble.)

If you don't believe that feeling attractive is a big issue for women, then test it out by forgetting to comment when your partner buys some new clothes or goes to the hairdresser. Better still, tell her she wasted her money and the hairstyle doesn't suit her. Then watch what happens for the next few days.

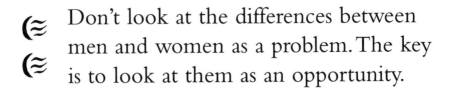

Don't look at the differences between men and women as a problem. The key is to look at them as an opportunity.

When I bring flowers home for Diane, when I support her buying what she needs, when I help her shop for a dress, when I tell her I love her again and again, even though she already knows it, I see her feminine beauty light up. Her joy empowers me and I feel good every time.

You can choose to see difference as an opportunity rather than as a problem, a possibility for you both to win and feel good in your relationship.

TELL ME YOU LOVE ME

When a woman says, "Tell me you love me," avoid saying stupid things like, "You already know it, I married you and I'm still with you." That makes sense to you, and any guy would agree your partner should already know it. But that is not what a woman wants to hear. Remember, she is an alien; unlike you, she wants to hear again and again that you love her. Many women don't think of telling you that they would like more loving attention because they assume you know that already. They forget that your needs are often different.

Instead of telling you what her needs are your partner will sometimes get upset and you won't know why! Next thing you are both in conflict, feeling disconnected, and you don't even know why. Tell her that you love her. Yes, again! Watch her reaction. Your partner needs to know that you are still attracted to her, that you still love her. I challenge you to exhaust the number of times you can tell her this. Don't only say it in words; say it in the way you touch her, with flowers, by phoning during the day. Think of creative ways of letting her know you love her.

IF YOU ARE SINGLE

If you are single and courting, don't forget to let a woman know, in as many ways as you can, that you are attracted to her. Be aware of the type of energy you are sending out. If you are attracted to a woman at a party but she doesn't respond and turns her back or gives you the message to leave, it isn't necessarily because she doesn't like feeling attractive, it more likely has to do with you. She could be looking for a different sort of man.

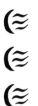 If you want women to be interested in you, you may need to develop your appearance, your health and fitness, your personality, and, not least of all, your self-awareness.

In the 1970s I spent two years traveling the world. From Bali I traveled overland through Asia, India, and Europe, and I undertook many training programs in personal development. When I returned to Australia I had no trouble attracting relationships. When I started teaching "Mindpowers," a personal development course, many women showed interest in me. I had already attracted a wonderful woman, Diane, my wife now for many years, so I was not open to other relationships, but it was obvious at my seminars that the interest was there.

I suggest you do some self-development courses and read books about how to open your heart to a woman and how to make love. There are numerous personal development courses that will teach you how to give and receive love.

Once you have developed a relationship with a woman you love, never negate her attractiveness or you may lose her and never know why. Don't talk about the attractiveness of other women in front of your partner if you want her to stay with you. If she feels that she is no longer attractive to you then she won't feel great about your relationship!

Once you have been with your partner for a period of time and she sees the possibility of your spending the rest of your lives together, she will carry out all sorts of tests to see if you are the right one. Even when you are married she will continue to carry out these tests, mostly unconsciously, because this behavior is instinctive.

THE PANDA BEAR TEST

I often tell a story to men in seminars—while Diane is elsewhere with the women describing us men as aliens and explaining how to relate to us. The story always brings insight as well as great amusement. It is the story of the mating of the panda bear. I first heard this analogy at More University.

When the female panda bear comes into heat she fights the male because she wants to see if he is the right one. She claws, she scratches, she bites. If he gives up and goes away another panda bear soon arrives.

The female continues to fight until she attracts the strongest panda bear. Only then will she mate. It's survival of the fittest.

This panda bear behavior occurs with humans, but it's obviously carried out in a much more sophisticated manner. Watch your woman after you have been partners for a period of time and notice her testing you. She "scratches," "claws," and "bites" to see if you are fit enough to be her partner. You might recognize the panda bear in your woman.

The silent treatment is an example of this. Your partner will tell you there is nothing the matter when obviously there is. This is "scratching." Then she starts the "clawing," which includes slamming doors or smashing dishes. There are more socialized forms of scratching and clawing, but they are still panda bear tactics.

If all this fails then finally she "bites" by leaving home or sleeping in the spare bedroom for a few days. That is a bite that really hurts a guy, especially when he has no idea what he has done, or it seems so insignificant that he cannot understand why she is so upset.

He tries to explain his side of the story, telling her not to feel as she does. Believe me, she will never say: "Thank you for telling me not to feel like that." Her emotions do not hear the "logic" of the male, so you are wasting your time. Stop trying to give explanations and telling her how she should feel. She couldn't care less if your argument makes sense—all she knows is that she is hurt. Once she has scratched and clawed and bitten and all that has failed, eventually she may withhold sex completely, and that is the final bite. She wants you to be able to handle all that and still say: "I love you, I want to be with you, and I'm happy I married you." She is conducting a panda bear test to see if you are the strongest and best bear. Once you understand her motives, it will really help you to stay sane and handle all that feminine energy.

Are you a big enough bear to handle all that? This is the question to ask yourself. Or should you run off and let someone else be her mate? Go ahead, call her names and leave, but let me tell you something: you will only find another panda bear when you meet another woman. She may have a different way of scratching and biting, but it will still occur. It might not happen in the early stages of your relationship,

but as you get closer and more intimate she will do her panda bear test,
I guarantee.

KALI, WILD VERSION OF THE PANDA BEAR

Hindu mythology has helped me deal with Diane's panda bear. In this
mythology, the goddess Kali depicts the fierce warrior energy a woman
shows when she needs to protect something she holds dear. Modern
women's groups speak of the many goddess aspects within every woman.
When you see a woman nurturing another you are meeting the Greek
goddess Demeter; when you see her sensual side you meet Aphrodite;
and when you see her intuitive side there is Persephone.

Kali, the Goddess of Protection, is depicted in Hindu paintings with
a sword in one hand, a man's severed head in the other, and her foot on
the corpse of her lover, Shiva. Kali looks like a wild version of the panda
bear. However, although she looks wild she is the Goddess of Protection, and inevitably Kali will surface as a woman gets closer and closer
to you.

Kali is especially likely to appear during a heightened state of sexual pleasure, when your partner is surrendering to a deeper level of
orgasm than she has ever experienced before. She can become frightened and resist because she is not certain if she trusts you enough to
surrender totally. Women resist this form of surrender because their
power has been subdued by male domination for more than two thousand years. To surrender totally, to orgasm at a level where she has never
been before with you, requires a lot of trust.

When going into the unknown Kali may appear, and you could
have a wild woman on your hands. You need to be a conscious, wise
man, skilled in the art of lovemaking, to handle Kali. So when she
appears, recognize her; when panda bear appears, recognize her. Realize
that they appear when a woman needs to trust you, when she wants
more assurance of your love, more attention, more recognition, more
affection. Love her, be with her, give her reason to trust you in the
future. Don't put her down, do not abandon her or make her feel bad.

UNDERSTANDING FEMALE TENSION

An important secret to understand about women is that, because they are capable of reproduction, they are generators of enormous energy. In the courses she conducts Diane tells women that their ovaries are power packs and can be a constant source of energy when they learn to acknowledge this energy and direct it. Being a man, I don't know what it feels like carrying that sort of reproductive energy around.

This natural generation and buildup of reproductive energy in women can create tension that comes out in bursts of energy, such as anger, yelling, or crying, or in totally inexplicable behavior over something apparently insignificant. Some men take the brunt of any outburst and start thinking, "She's crazy, why did I marry her?" because they don't understand.

Women often don't understand why they are so tense. After an outburst they usually become calm again and may apologize. This syndrome, often most noticeable just before menstruation, is commonly called premenstrual tension or premenstrual syndrome (PMS).

This buildup of energy can manifest in different forms for different women. For some it shows up as depression (often the result of suppressed outbursts), while other women express it by being sexually turned on. What's important to understand is that men very often reflect their woman's tense energy. It's like magnetic induction. Often your partner doesn't even have to say anything—you just pick it up from being around her. It is important for you to recognize this when it happens and, instead of focusing only on trying to reduce your own tension, learn ways to calm each other down. One pleasant way to reduce this buildup of energy is having a good orgasm. When a woman is in her sexiest time of the month it can sometimes take four or five orgasms a day to release this energy. That's why it is important to have many lovemaking skills.

In 1987 Diane and I lived in a house in California for a couple of weeks. It was part of More University, where people were studying sexuality and practicing extended orgasm every day. Some of the advanced students had assignments where they had to sexually pleasure each other five to ten times per day. There must have been twenty people living in that house and I have never met a more relaxed, contented group.

Orgasm is not the only way to reduce this buildup of energy. Holding your partner tight and giving her lots of attention in other ways can also calm her energy.

Next time you notice your partner is starting to get tense, give her lots of attention and lots of hugging before it gets out of control. Take her out and indulge her with a little wine, dinner, dancing, and hugging throughout the night, and complete it with a good lovemaking session. You will be well on the way to a more harmonious relationship and a much better sex life. If your woman is aware of this energy she generates, that is great because you can simply ask her if she is feeling tension. She may say, "I'm feeling really tight and need loving now," in which case you can either have a lovemaking session, make time for her to honor herself sexually, or give her a strong, firm hug and don't let go until the tension has gone.

BEAUTY IS . . .

Your perception of beauty almost certainly has been conditioned by the media. The body that you think of as typically beautiful is not the body that was regarded as beautiful years ago. For example, Rubens painted large, voluptuous women because, to the people of his era, that shape was beautiful. Popular models of today would not have rated in those days. Today in countries such as India a slim woman is still not considered beautiful. It is possible to perceive beauty differently.

Peter, a participant in one of our workshops, told us, "I'm attracted to women who are round and soft. To me they are more womanly. I like my woman to be soft and shapely. To feel the shape of her hips on top of me when we are making love is magnificent, and to feel the softness of her tummy when I'm on top always turns me on."

Diane commented: "If you don't feel like Peter about more rounded women and your partner isn't as thin as when you first met, you can reeducate yourself to change your focus. What is your partner's skin like? her hair? her lips? her eyes? Tell her the things about her body that you like. 'It turns me on when I kiss your knees or your thighs. You are such a sexy woman and I love you.'"

Tell her only things that you like. It's like the old song—accentuate the positive, eliminate the negative, and don't mess with "Mr. In-Between." Your partner has probably been conditioned not to like some parts of her body and will not believe you if you tell her they are beautiful and that you like them. She probably doesn't think her yoni is attractive, but she is not sure. So you, as an extraordinary lover, have an opportunity to tell her how beautiful her yoni is—how you love its color, its scent, its softness.

Seventy out of one hundred women in a recent workshop said they were concerned about the scent of their yoni. Give your partner positive affirmation about her fragrance. If you don't like the scent, then don't mention it. The scent of the yoni can be affected by diet; meat, for example, gives it a stronger scent. It is the same with your semen; diet affects the taste.

AVOID GOING TOO FAR TOO SOON

In that same workshop John said: "Kathy, my first wife, was an excellent panda bear and especially good at yelling and withholding sex. I want to know what to do when women do that."

Another participant, Mark, said: "Yes, that's what I want to know as well. One night when I was pleasuring my wife she couldn't orgasm and she became violent. Her eyes looked wild. She really didn't look like herself. She started crying hysterically, and when I tried to comfort her, she yelled: 'Don't touch me!' I got the full strength of her panda bear, or maybe it was Kali? Whoever it was it frightened me."

Mark told me the full story. He had been pleasuring his wife, Joanne, for more than an hour; each time she came to a point of orgasm he stopped, and once she was calmed he started pleasuring her again. He had repeated this about ten times.

Mark had taken things too far.

Women sometimes reach a space where they're too stimulated to come. They cannot let go of all the energy because they don't trust their partner enough to allow themselves to be so much out of control. So it's important to avoid going too far. Find out what works best for your partner.

When a woman is on the edge of going into a higher space than she has ever been before, Kali can appear. Kali comes up for protection and when Kali (or the panda bear) come up, be aware of what is happening. Don't try to rationalize or argue, whatever you do. Instead, show her your strength by staying with her. Be there totally for her and tell her you love her. If she yells abuse at you, let it pass. It's important to allow her to express her feelings.

When women turn on their panda bear what they often want most is attention. However, most of the time they don't know how evil and mean they look; if only they could see themselves at this time! How can they expect anyone to come near them? Awareness on both your parts is essential to overcome these situations.

Remember that Kali appears when your woman trusts you more than ever before and is on the edge of reaching new realms of pleasure with herself and with you.

This is a great affirmation of her love for you, so think of it as the panda bear test to see if you still love her. The easiest way out of a situation like this is to say: "I can't live with you any more," and walk out. Even though you may feel that is what you want to do, try to pause and see beyond this. Imagine this moment as a gift, an opportunity for your relationship to reach even deeper levels. Understand that once you show her you will not run away she will trust you more in the future. Think of it in this way: the best panda bear wins, and this woman has the best panda bear—you—an extraordinary lover.

A WOMAN LIKES A MAN

Over the past decade more and more men have become conscious of the need to be in touch with their feminine side. Men and women are no longer bound by the old roles of sexual stereotypes; the notions of macho man and submissive wife are outdated.

At the same time many women have developed their competitive, directed, and assertive side while many men have cultivated their feeling, intimate, and relational side. This is a positive step. However, taken to the extreme without consciously being aware of the dynamics in your relationship, it can create problems. A lot of women now complain that men are no longer "men," that they like a man who is confident, clear, and decisive, particularly when it comes to making a commitment in relationship, someone who can show her a love that she can trust in, even when she is upset and "doing her panda bear."

Listen to Keith's story.

"In my twenties and early thirties I was in touch with my male energy. I was directed, focused, and on a mission to make things happen. I started my own business in event management. Then, through listening to some personal development speakers, I started to expand my ideas on what it is to be a man. I met Judy, my current partner, and she encouraged me—or rather, insisted—that I develop more of the emotional, intimate, reflective side of myself, my feminine side. I read numerous books, took vegetarian cooking classes, had frequent massages, and gave up competitive sports to do weekend workshops on personal discovery. I became the popular, sensitive, New Age guy I had read about. Then, through a series of circumstances, I lost my business and had even more time to explore my emotional side.

"After being with Judy now for nearly three years she often complains that I am not focused or decisive enough and she doesn't feel supported by me. She tells me about other successful guys at her work. I feel criticized and hurt. Our sex life is not as passionate either."

Keith came to see me to ask for some advice.

I first acknowledged his efforts to develop his feminine side, and it sounded as if Judy was well in touch with her masculine side. Her career in real estate was obviously successful, and she was taking charge of their financial situation and their relationship in general. They had certainly progressed from the stereotype "I'm the man and you're the woman" of their parents' generation. However, they had fallen into another stereotype, that of the New Age, "sensitive guy, powerful woman." This stereotype can be just as restrictive if you don't realize what is happening and you become identified with those new roles.

Something else that can happen is if you have equal masculine and feminine qualities and your partner has equal masculine and feminine qualities, then in bed the polarity between you is neutralized and the sexual attraction is not as powerful. What was once passionate sex between opposite poles becomes lukewarm lovemaking between equals.

In order to re-create the fire and the powerful attraction between men and women we need to play with our roles and let go of the cultural ideal of what we "should" be. We need to determine what is needed in our professional life and what is needed in bed in order to get what we want, and then draw on the appropriate male or female side of our nature from one situation to another. In sexual loving this might require a woman to let down her guard, forego her resistances, and open up to being madly, truly, and deeply loved; then to connect with the goddess of love and sensuality within her, allowing the beauty of her feminine radiance to shine through. For you it may mean you need to tap more in to your masculine side so she can feel your strength, directedness, and confidence, and especially your presence and passion.

Your partner might be a successful career woman and you may often feel overpowered by her or in competition for power, but there is a big chance that in her heart of hearts she still wants to be cherished and honored as a goddess, "to feel your yearning to enrapture her with your love." This comes not from a need in you for sexual satisfaction or power or control, but from a burning desire to have a deep, passionate, heartfelt connection with the person you love.

After explaining this to Keith and Judy in a subsequent consultation, I suggested the first thing they could try is to playfully explore the idea of taking on the roles of Shiva and Shakti in a tantric ritual, such as the one I suggested earlier in this chapter: making a devotion to each other before making love, and then looking for the Shakti and Shiva within each other. That way they could step out of their predictable roles for a time and become the God and Goddess of Love. This is an excellent way to bring back some polarity and passion and to nurture one of your woman's deepest needs in the dance of sexual loving: to feel your masculine love in intimate union with her sacred, feminine essence.

I am not suggesting you shouldn't develop your more sensitive, emotional side. Women love a man who they can be emotional and intimate with. This is an important part of tantra, to be able to open your heart and turn sex in to making love. However, in cultivating your female side be careful not to lose touch with certain aspects of your masculine nature. When you find yourself becoming indecisive, non-committal, out of touch with any direction or vision, and unable to feel your sexual virility in bed, it's time to regroup and build new confidence in your male expression.

You have the ability to be in touch with your feelings and at the same time to embrace your male essence when you need it. The key lies in being able to be free to develop and access what is required at different times and, even more specifically, from moment to moment. Then in your lovemaking you will be able to give your woman more of whatever she needs, both physically and emotionally. You will feel confident in your love. A man with "spine" and an open heart is very attractive to a woman.

3

Heartfelt Loving

When Diane and I have asked groups of women in our workshops what they would like more of in lovemaking, they have shared many things. The most common things women want are more romance, intimacy, and love, and for their men to be more in touch with their own feelings. These are all concerned with opening the heart. The more you know about how to touch your woman's heart the more sexually responsive she will be.

Women are more open to lovemaking through the heart than through the yoni because of the way they are created physically and energetically and due to social conditioning.

Physically the female genitals are inside the body, so a lot of the sexual energy is inside and harder to awaken, slower to warm. Generally it takes a woman more foreplay than it does for a man to become sexually aroused. The male genitals are outside the body, so the sexual energy is more external and easier to excite. In the heart center, the area of intimacy, the opposite situation occurs. Here, men are usually more inward and women more outward. It is generally easier for a woman to be more intimate than a man. This may not be the case in your relationship, but most of the time this is the way it is.

Next time you're at a social gathering take note of what the groups of men talk about and what the groups of women talk about. You will find most men talk about situations and events, whereas women talk about their feelings about those events. Women are more ready to be intimate. This is related to social conditioning. We learn as we are growing up how to be a man or a woman and how we are to behave. In our society men are acknowledged for having a strong sexual drive. A lot of young men like to tell their friends how many women they have slept with and how well they satisfied those women. Men are supposed to be sexy, hard, and ready to go all night, and they are acknowledged for it.

In contrast, young women, when they first feel their sexual energy, are encouraged to suppress it; they are not to show it. If they act on it they risk being labeled a "bad girl." Young men often like to let everyone know they are having sex, but young women tend to keep it quiet because they are supposed to be "good."

Times are changing. Pop singer Madonna clearly promotes that being sexy is powerful, but conditioning still exists deep in women's subconscious. A man wants to marry a "good girl," but once he is married he wants her to love sex. One moment a woman is revered as a virgin and the next she is asked to be multiorgasmic. In our workshops we focus on the fact that "good girls" do it and they thoroughly love it. In this way we start healing negative programming about women's sexuality and about a woman's desire to be and feel sexy.

At an early age you were probably told: "Big boys don't cry. Your friends will think you are weak," or "Grow up, son. Don't speak to your father like that." In other words: "Shut up and don't express your feelings." Later on in your relationship your wife might say: "Tell me how you feel about me, John." A common reply is: "I love you, of course. I married you, didn't I?" Now that is about as intimate as some guys get and it's not entirely their fault. They have been conditioned by society that to be a "real man" they must suppress their feelings.

Although men often proclaim how different they are from their fathers, it is interesting to observe how often these unconscious patterns of behavior arise. In one workshop a man told of how he had caught himself doing this. When his son felt sad or upset he would always distract the boy. "Let's go to the beach," or "Let's watch football." The man thought he was doing a great job by distracting the child until Diane pointed out to him that, by trying to change his son's feelings, he was basically saying to the child that it was not okay for him to feel as he did. By distracting the boy he forced him to suppress his feelings and bottle them up.

> (≈
> (≈
> (≈
> (≈
> (≈
> (≈
> (≈
> In your relationship you can play a vital role in awakening your beloved's sexual energy. One of the most powerful ways you can do this is through the heart, by opening more to intimacy. However, it's often just as difficult for men to be intimate as it is for women to be sexy, because to be a real man you are not supposed to show too much intimacy.

A better way would be to sit down with his son and say: "Tom, how are you feeling?" Initially Tom might not say anything, but if the father stays with him for a while the boy might respond. He might say that he's okay or he might say he's feeling sad. The father could let him talk further while not saying much at all, or he could ask his son to share his story with him. As the boy shares his story he should be allowed to do all the talking. Instead of saying, "You shouldn't feel like that," or "This is the way to do it," it is better for the father to simply empathize with what his son is feeling: "I understand that you feel sad (angry, annoyed, etc.) and it's okay." The father might relate a similar experience he had. By listening to what his father says, the boy can empathize with him and this will help him feel better about his own situation.

Remember, we must not place blame on our parents for our inability to express our feelings or show intimacy. In most cases our parents did the best they could with the knowledge and the conditioning they had at the time. In my parents' time it was expected that a man—the John Wayne type—would be in control of everything, including women and his feelings. Perhaps that image has been subconsciously imprinted in men to such an extent that we do not talk about our hurts or fears because this means we have lost control. However, women often interpret our lack of intimacy as coldness in the heart, and the colder she feels we are in the heart, the colder she becomes sexually in response.

Often in a relationship the woman doesn't want to make love because she's not getting enough attention or enough intimacy. Then, because she doesn't want sexual contact with her partner, he pulls away even further emotionally. He becomes less intimate. She then grows even less inclined to make love. And so it goes on.

If this continues long enough there is a strong chance this couple is heading for divorce. Once you are aware that your woman wants intimacy and romance and once she realizes that by refusing sex she will never receive your intimacy, you can both begin to do something about it.

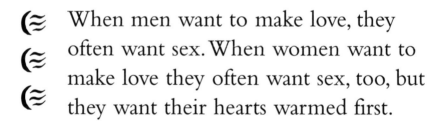

When men want to make love, they often want sex. When women want to make love they often want sex, too, but they want their hearts warmed first.

The more you help your woman to feel a heart connection with you, the more likely she will be to open up her sexual energy to you. This dynamic works in reverse for men. I know for myself the more Diane opens up her sexual energy to me the more love I feel. When she closes off her sexual energy I don't feel as close to her. This is because the way to a man's heart is through the yoni while the way to a woman's yoni is through the heart. To be intimate means to be in touch with and show more of my innermost feelings—intimacy equals in-to-me-see. Some men believe they will become much more intimate and loving when they meet the right partner. What they do not realize is that intimacy and the ability to send and receive love need to be developed within themselves. They do not realize that searching outside themselves is not the way to feel more love. Even though they already may have had many partners, they still believe that one day the right one will appear and that with her, all the love, intimacy, and romance will somehow magically occur.

What is important is to work on yourself first. This does not mean that you will not be able to find a woman who opens your heart more than others, but that is all a woman can do—trigger your heart to feel more intimate. She cannot actually create the feeling for you.

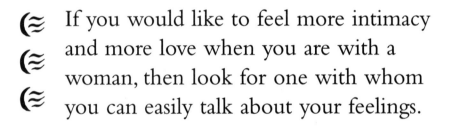 If you would like to feel more intimacy and more love when you are with a woman, then look for one with whom you can easily talk about your feelings.

I bet you often meet women like this but do not recognize them as women with whom you could be in a loving relationship, because in your search to find a beloved you are very likely looking for the "model" type. Like many men, you probably have been so seduced by the media that what you are looking for, deep down in your fantasies, is the Hollywood model with a near-perfect body, perfect hair, perfect looks, sexy, and, of course, only wanting you. So in your search for the right woman with whom to share your life you are looking for these superficial qualities rather than the triggering of your heart. One day you may meet the woman who most closely matches your media-like image and that is the one you settle for. Unfortunately, you often overlook the women who are much more loving and with whom you feel comfortable, the women with whom you laugh and in whom you confide.

GETTING IN TOUCH WITH
YOUR FEELINGS

I cannot emphasize too much how important it is for you to get in touch with your feelings if you want a better sex life.

There are many ways to learn to open up your heart and get in touch with your feelings. One such way is through rebirthing. Rebirthing takes the form of a continuous breathing session that can make you aware of deep feelings within you. Several years ago I took some sessions with a couple who are very experienced and extremely loving and supportive in their approach to rebirthing. It was one of the best things I have done in opening myself more to love. However, I would not advise you to go in to rebirthing lightly. If you are undertaking a rebirthing session it is important that you trust and feel comfortable with the person guiding you. You must also be clear about why you are doing it.

Another way to connect with your feelings is to be aware of the way you say things. In your conversations with people you are close to, instead of saying: "I think . . ." say, "I feel . . ." For example, the phrase "I think the section on lovemaking as a meditation was . . ." is probably easy for you to complete. However, the statement "The section on lovemaking as a meditation made me feel . . ." is a little more difficult for most men. Try it for yourself! Men tend to focus on their conception and opinion of things rather than on their feelings about things. To become more intimate it is essential to become more in touch with your feelings.

Next time your partner does something that annoys you, instead of going in to reasons why she should not do something or telling her what to do, say: "When you do that, it makes me feel angry (insecure, resentful, etc.)." You are not blaming her, you are just honoring your feelings by telling her how you are feeling at the time. Even if she verbally retaliates, just say: "I'm telling you how I feel because I love you and you are the one I trust the most to share my feelings with," and leave it at that. Although she may be too angry to speak to you at the time she will hear you on her emotional level, and there is a good chance she will soften the next time she speaks to you.

Whenever you are stuck in expressing your feelings, breathe deeply, let go, and try again. "I'm feeling . . ." Keep breathing as you are expressing your feelings. When you feel blocked and you cannot identify what the feeling is, just breathe and you will find it will come much more easily to you.

One way that we blocked our feelings as children was to hold our breath. Watch children who are upset hold their breath and clench their teeth. Once they let the breath go they cry or scream and this allows them to feel again. Once you are in touch with your feelings and your heart is more open to romance, you will increase your intimacy with others.

HOW TO CREATE MORE INTIMACY

When you want to keep something hidden from someone you avoid eye contact. People who are not comfortable with eye contact are often afraid of others seeing something within that they don't want them to see—maybe it's secrets, or guilt, or a hidden shyness, or anger, or fear.

To develop intimacy, start looking into people's eyes for longer than you normally do while conversing with them. Doing this for too long can be intrusive, so do it with care and sensitivity. However, with people you trust, such as your partner, take the opportunity to open more to truth and allow them to see into you more.

MAKING EYE CONTACT

Sit or lie opposite each other while keeping eye contact. This is not a staring competition, but simply an opportunity to be more open, to allow yourself to be seen. Let your breathing be deep and continuous but try not to touch or hug. Your mind will be saying all sorts of things but they are just thoughts, so let them go like clouds passing across your mind. This is called thought release.

Each time you hold your breath you block off feelings and allow yourself to not be seen. Continue to release the breath throughout the process while checking into your heart center. How do you feel? If you feel uncomfortable that's okay. Do not try to fight it. It's a natural occurrence as you move toward becoming more intimate. It is all part of moving into the unknown.

After five minutes of no talking, with just breathing and eye contact, you can complete the exercise with a deep hug and talk about the experience. Try to share how it made you feel rather than talking about any concepts you may have regarding the process.

COMMUNICATING WHAT YOU ENJOY

Now start to communicate intimately with your partner. You could start with "What I like about making love with you is . . ." and complete the sentence. Then say it again. "What I like about making love with you is. . ." and say it again. For example:

"What I like about making love with you is the way you look into my eyes and make me feel loved."
"What I like about making love with you is getting the feeling that you are so close to me and trust me so much that you allow me to enter your body."
"What I like about making love with you is . . ."

If you run out of things to say and nothing else comes to mind, simply repeat: "What I like about making love with you is . . ." and something may come out that will surprise you or your partner. Through spontaneity, hidden truths may emerge. Your partner simply says, "thank you" every time you share something new.

This practice goes on for up to five minutes. If you reach a stage where you are totally uncomfortable and cannot find anything else to say, then experience that feeling of awkwardness because it is breaking through to another level of intimacy for you. Say it again: "What I like about making love with you is . . ." until the five minutes are up. Be careful not to get into discussions—this is a trust exercise that works on the premise that one person is allowed to speak the truth without the other interrupting. Maintain eye contact and keep breathing through the entire exchange.

In this practice it is very important to follow the structure. If you break the structure then the practice itself will likely not work, and you will have wasted your time doing it.

It is important to share what you like in lovemaking because often during lovemaking you expect your partner to behave in certain ways and you get upset when she doesn't, but you do not actually tell her how you might like her to be. You may get annoyed when she does certain things, but you don't tell her because you don't want to upset her; you don't want to rock the boat. So you go on feeling annoyed because you are not getting what you want or because she does something that upsets you. The same thing happens for her. This frustration shows in your lovemaking. If you have enough trust between you, it's best to share these frustrations away from your time of lovemaking.

The next practice enters into an area of relationship where very few people venture. Here one partner can tell the absolute truth while the other person just listens without comment.

It does not mean you are blaming your partner and it does not mean your partner has to change according to what you want. This is breaking through to a deep level of intimacy and requires an enormous amount of trust. That trust will then carry over into your lovemaking and you will find you will go to much deeper levels once you trust a person this much.

If you wish to progress to a level of relationship that is extraordinary, then you need to be able to share the things you like and dislike about your relationship.

COMMUNICATING WHAT YOU DON'T ENJOY

Continue the practice as outlined above, this time using the words "What I don't like about making love with you is . . ." Remember to breathe, especially when you get stuck. Breathe with your partner when she is stuck.

"What I don't like about making love with you is that I always have to instigate the lovemaking."

"What I don't like about making love with you is that you never get on top without me asking you to."

"What I don't like about making love with you is how you always get up and go to the bathroom during our lovemaking or after our lovemaking."

"What I don't like about making love with you is . . ."

And you continue. Your partner simply says, "thank you" after each statement and realizes that all you are doing is telling the truth and that she does not have to do anything about it. She is just allowing you the truth. If she starts arguing with you or defending herself, then what she is saying is, "I don't want to hear the truth. Keep secrets from me." But if she is there totally, she affirms her unconditional love for you. "Not only will I love you when everything is right, but I will love you no matter what."

After five minutes your partner commences: "What I don't like about making love with you is . . ." and you must remember to say "thank you" every time she shares something with you.

After you've both spoken, do not enter into any communication. Hold your partner's hands and, while keeping eye contact, breathe in and say to yourself, "I am loved," and absorb that. Even though you might be reacting to something she said, the truth is that you are loved—you are loved so much that your partner has shared the truth with you and she trusted you to hear it. As you breathe in, say to yourself, "I am loved" and absorb that through your entire being. Absorb the energy of "I am loved" through your hands and breathe it up to your chest and heart region. Try to feel that you are loved in your heart.

As you let go of the breath, send your heart energy through your hands into your beloved as you say, "I love you." Send and receive as much love as you can. Say to yourself: "I am loved" as you breathe in and "I love you" as you breathe out.

Continue this practice for a few minutes, then both gently shut your eyes. Place your hands over your heart center (the area in the middle of your chest, level with your breasts) with your right hand on top of your left hand, and mentally take the breath to that area to open to as much love as you can feel. Do this again for several minutes. During this time take moments to gently open your eyes and look at your partner and feel the privilege of having someone whom you can trust and with whom you can share on this level. Really try to appreciate this great gift, remembering that many people do not have someone to love or someone from whom to receive love.

≈ ≈ ≈ ≈ You need to learn to send more love to your partner through your hands, through your touch, through your lingam, through your eyes, and through what you say, and at the same time learn to receive as much love as you can from your partner.

Next, with eyes open and either sitting or standing, press your heart centers firmly together in a deep embrace. Yab-yum is a great position to adopt because the body's energy centers for the heart and sexual center are joined simultaneously. Yab-yum can also be done with the man's legs stretched straight out, or it is even easier if the man sits on a chair and the woman sits on top. While sitting in yab-yum feel your connectedness again. While eye-gazing you might say to each other something like, "I love you. I enjoyed that exploration and I'd like to do it again sometime."

This practice could take half an hour, but I promise you it will be half an hour well worth the effort, even if you only do it once. If you wish, you can again share how it felt for you. Share feelings only; don't have an intellectual discussion. You may wish to enter into lovemaking afterward. Do whatever is appropriate at the time.

If you do this exercise with a person with whom you are not in a permanent relationship, use the statements: "What I enjoy about making love is . . ." and "What I don't enjoy about making love is . . ." This is letting the other person know your boundaries, and it will certainly save a lot of mind reading. It is best to have clear communication from the beginning.

If you burst into laughter during the exercise, don't worry about it. You might just laugh at the unusualness of it, but keep doing it anyway. Go into this practice with an attitude that you are opening new ways

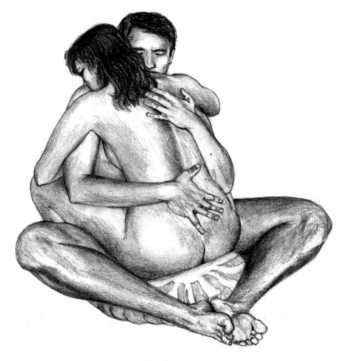

YAB-YUM

to connect with your partner. Sometimes you will find that your laughter will turn into tears; again, that is just a natural way the body frees up
energy. Honor all your emotions as they emerge throughout the exercise. Allowing all of you to be seen is part of being an exciting, emotive
human being.

As you become familiar with this exercise you can use either eye
contact, breathing, or the kind of sharing practiced in this exercise as
foreplay before lovemaking to guide you into a deeper connection with
one another.

When you first start these intimacy exercises it might feel awkward,
but as you practice it becomes easier and a natural thing to do. On the
one hand you are afraid to tell the truth about your feelings because you
feel that level of truth will hurt your partner, but on the other hand
your whole relationship suffers if you do not tell the truth. Remember,
hiding things from your partner intensifies those negative feelings and

fears. Sharing brings negative feelings to the surface and disempowers them. This makes more energy available for bonding. This process of sharing your deep feelings is a great opportunity to expand not only your intimacy and your relationship, but also your ability to go deeper into lovemaking, into letting your sexual ecstasy develop.

Hal and Rosie had been going out for about six months when they participated in one of our seminars. During one of these intimacy sessions they repeated to each other "One of my fears about sexuality is. . ." These are some of the things they shared.

Hal said:

- "One of my fears about sexuality is that my penis is not big enough."
- "One of my fears is that Rosie will make love with someone else."
- "One of my fears about sexuality is that I will get AIDS."
- "One of my fears is that I'll ejaculate too soon."

It is valuable for you to mentally list a few fears yourself while reading this. Simply say to yourself, "One of my fears about sexuality is . . ." and see what comes up.

Rosie said:

- "One of my fears about sexuality is that my breasts are not big enough."
- "One of my fears is that my body is not attractive."
- "One of my fears about sexuality is that I won't have an orgasm."
- "One of my fears is that Hal will leave me."
- "One of my fears about sexuality is that my vagina smells bad."

Dillan and Rebecca had been in a committed relationship for five years; with the eye-gazing exercise they shared a peak experience in their sex life. Dillan said: "The sexual experience I really enjoyed with you was when . . ." and he described the whole sexual experience. Rebecca said "thank you," and then she shared her experience.

This is a great way to learn what your partner really enjoys. You can take a few of these things and integrate them into your lovemaking. You may have forgotten some of those things that, at different times, turned your partner on so much.

When next you have some private time with your lover, or even during dinner, instead of your usual conversation say: "I'd like to play a game with you if you're willing." Then quickly describe the structure and begin. "Some of the things I like about you are . . ." This is a good one to get things started. Then say: "Okay, now it's your turn." This could lead to more intimate sharing, like the exercise suggested above, either at that moment or at a later date. Try this with a woman you have not been dating for very long. She will remember her night out with you and see you as an interesting person. Anyone can be ordinary but, remember, you can be an extraordinary lover.

When you are sharing intimate feelings with your wife things may emerge that are best not discussed at the time, especially if you react negatively. My advice is to leave your discussion at least until the next day. Give yourself time to integrate the information and lessen any negative emotional charge the words may have had on you, because it is important to understand the real purpose of this practice—it is not to blame your partner or to off-load garbage on her, but to open up to more intimacy, more truth, and deeper lovemaking.

My experience after doing exercises like this is that, during lovemaking, my heart is much more open, and so having sex turns into another vibration where passion and intimacy are harmoniously interwoven.

TALK

To encourage more intimacy you need to talk more during lovemaking. In our survey about what women would like more of in lovemaking many said they would like their men to whisper things to them. But for men it is often difficult to think of what to say. You cannot repeat "I love you" throughout a whole lovemaking session, but you can learn different ways of saying it. A lot of men shut their eyes and get lost in their own space while making love. Women, too, get lost in their own space, and when this happens the sex can be more like mutual masturbation than making love. For more intimacy to occur you have to learn to express any sexy or loving thoughts that come into your mind instead of just thinking them. However, it is important to realize that sometimes things you say might be misinterpreted. Men and women are different and they hear things differently.

In one of our seminars I mentioned to Alex about talking more during lovemaking and he tried it the next time he was making love. When he saw his lover's nipples protruding he said, "You are responding really well," but she didn't seem to like that comment. Later, when they had finished making love, he thought to himself "She's really good." So he said: "Sarah, you are really good." He thought he had done well saying that, because he normally did not say anything—lots of "oohs!" and "aahs!" but no speaking. The next day at the seminar Sarah expressed her appreciation of his efforts to talk to her, but she hated what he'd said. The other women in the group agreed. The men looked dumbfounded!

Why were the women turned off by what Alex had said? Because women need their attractiveness—not their functionalism—recognized and praised. Alex's comments were about getting it right. It may appeal to a man to hear "You are good"; to him it means that he is good in bed and that is great. But generally such comments are a turn-off for a woman. What she hears is "good."

"Good compared to whom? Responding well? I'm not an object!" is her response.

The men then asked: "Well what do you want to hear?" So we invited the women to write down what they would like men to say to them during lovemaking. They agreed to do this on the condition that

the men wrote down what they would like women to say during lovemaking as well. We collated the responses and the results were amaz-
ingly different. Here are some of the things women wrote.

- "Your fragrance is like jasmine."
- "I'm your lover forever."
- "I love the feel of your skin; it's so soft, like satin."
- "You have the most beautiful . . ."
- "It's wonderful to be inside you."
- "You're sending shivers up and down my spine."
- "I love the shape of your breasts; they feel like Heaven in
  my hands."
- "You're a very sensuous woman."
- "I enjoy the pleasure of your passion."
- "I love your yoni's perfume."

What the men wanted to hear were things such as:

- "More, more, I want you to come deeper inside me."
- "You feel so big inside me."
- "You're the best."
- "Your lingam is so hot."

The women laughed at what the men wanted them to say. They could
not believe it. Meanwhile, the men looked a bit confused about what the
women wanted them to say. So for an interesting exercise you could ask
your beloved to write down what she would like to hear and you write
down what you would like to hear and give it to each other to read.

Even if these comments do not sound important to you, learn to
say them anyway during lovemaking. Don't be mute; be a great, romantic lover. You might think this is a little calculated, because romance
should be spontaneous. Yes, spontaneity is a wonderful ingredient, but if
your conversation in bed is simply, "I love you. Ooh! Ooh! Aah! That's
good!" that is not the vocabulary of a great lover. Learn to be a great

talker in bed. Practice saying wonderful things in your beloved's ear, things she wants to hear and not things you want to tell her.

I would like to offer some inspiration from ancient Hindu mythology, which contains many conversations between gods and goddesses: between Shiva and Shakti, Brahma and Saraswati, Vishnu and Laxshmi. Here are some interpretations from *The Tree of Ecstasy* by Dolores Ashcroft-Nowicki.

> Vishnu: How beautiful thou art, fair as a garden of fragrant flowers. Thou art an instrument of exquisite pleasure whose harmonies fill the universe with beauty. Nothing can surpass thee, thou art perfection.
>
> Laxshmi: Thou art the preserver of life. If I am the instrument of pleasure, then thine is the hand that plays the melody. No music is heard that comes not from our joining; without Vishnu and Laxshmi nothing will grow or prosper, and there will be no love and no fertility.

Here is a line from Brahma to Saraswati that I like.

> Saraswati, radiant being of my soul. Thou art together with me and we are one being.

Next time you are making love with your beloved, hold her in your arms as if you are one being, one person, one radiant light, and say something wonderful to her. Before you touch her sacred parts, her yoni or her breasts, say something romantic, honoring, and respectful. Here is what Brahma would say to Saraswati as he was about to kiss the yoni of his goddess in adoration.

> Thou art the seven ecstasies of union, thou art the holder of life. The singer of sweet songs. In union with thee my body becomes a temple of joy. Wrapped in the arms of Saraswati, Brahma knows only the infinite ecstasy of creation.

I assure you, this sounds better to her than "Ooh! Aah! I love you!" or just "Ooh! Aah!" You might feel uncomfortable with it at first, but persist because women love romance. Allow the romantic in you to come out and create your own tender words.

This is what Vishnu said to Laxshmi as he entered her.

> Lady of beauty, let me know thy sweetness. Let me touch the inner petals of thy sacred chakra with the lingam and fill the vase of life to overflowing. Thy hands are cool with scented oil and thy lips are warm with wine.

This is assuming that you have offered wine to your beloved and that you have massaged each other with scented oils as part of loveplay!

I like to use an adaptation from the following conversation between Shiva and Shakti.

"Diane, you are my precious one, my jewel, my incomparable lady of joy. Without you I would have no power in the world of men. Into your arms I place my body. Let me be your toy, my lady of perfume, my lady of sweet perfume."

You might take just one sentence from this if you like it and use it regularly. After a while it becomes a natural part of lovemaking, and women love it because it is romantic.

CREATE ROMANCE

An atmosphere of romance is always conducive to intimate lovemaking experiences, and women dearly love it. In creating the atmosphere, see yourself as a great lover and let your creative self step out of the ordinary and create something magical, something extraordinary.

Romance begins well before the first kiss. Men are often only romantic and hug and kiss when they are in bed. For women, romance starts much earlier. Foreplay to a man is kissing her neck and breasts. Foreplay to a woman can be a bunch of flowers or a phone call during the day telling her that you love her. If you are fortunate enough to have in your life a woman who loves you, I assure you that you cannot tell her too many times that you are madly in love with her. Ring her up many times before your planned evening. "I'm just calling to let you know that I love you and I'm really looking forward to our time together this evening." It's as simple as that. And remember to touch her throughout the day in a loving way, not just when you get into bed.

Neil, who took one of our classes, told Diane and me: "Although I consider myself a good lover, I realized after you talked about romance that rarely through the day do I kiss or hug my wife. I'm sure many days go by sometimes when we don't even touch. I love my wife very much, but I've fallen into the habit of not touching her unless it's during sex. So I decided to make it a practice that every time I heard Fay doing something in the kitchen I would go in and touch her on the upper back, give her a kiss, tell her something affirmative, and say, "I love you." It amazes me that such a simple thing has added so much to our love life again. What I've found is that I'm enthusiastic now about creating more ways to practice the art of romance every day. Fay knows I'm doing it because of what I've learned here in the workshop, but she still loves it."

Take on the image of being a great lover and devise ways to romance your woman. But remember that what is sexy and romantic to you may not be to her. For example, imagine your woman coming home from work before your planned night, rushing in the door, grabbing you on the genitals, smothering you in kisses, and saying, "I want you now. I'm going to give it all to you tonight. I can't wait." Sounds sexy, doesn't it? It does to a guy. However, if you did the same to her it could be a complete turn-off.

This might be hard to believe for anyone who hasn't lived with a woman, but that dialogue is the stuff of which movies are made—he grabs her breast and immediately she goes into ecstasy and starts ripping off his clothes. These movies are made by men, and sometimes by women who have been seduced by male sexuality and who have probably never had sex with someone skilled in the arts of romance or love-making.

In reality, telling your beloved that you're pleased to be spending time with her or bringing her flowers to show that you care for her will turn her on much more than grabbing her breasts.

A guy once said to me: "Why didn't God make men and women think the same? It would have saved a lot of messing around!" I reminded him that women often seem like aliens to men and that, although their needs sometimes do not make sense to us, we can still win at the lovemaking game by responding to them. A great lover will give his partner what turns her on, not what he thinks will turn her on. Give your partner breakfast in bed on the morning of your special evening, and when you come home bring a bottle of champagne.

My suggestion is to make a special time for this romantic meeting. Mark it on your calendar and set aside at least three hours. People often make the point that it's not romantic if it's planned. However, it is my experience that if you set a time it creates the opportunity for spontaneity to happen. There is nothing romantic about making love if the phone keeps ringing or the kids are screaming or running in and out of the room. Once you mark in your time on the calendar, you can organize it so the kids are out of the house, the phone is off the hook, and the doors are locked. It is especially important for busy couples to claim some time for this special happening. Busy couples, couples with families, or couples in business together often do not get to make love until late at night, and by that time they often do not want to think about anything except going to sleep. After years of this their lovemaking loses its juice, its excitement. They say: "Well, I can't afford the time!" That is ridiculous! May I point out that they find time to watch TV; they find time to go to the gym; they find the time to go jogging; they find time to read newspapers. It's simply that they have put love-making at the end of their priority list.

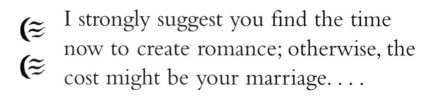 I strongly suggest you find the time now to create romance; otherwise, the cost might be your marriage. . . .

It is a ridiculous situation to put yourselves in. Look at your calendar—birthdays, social gatherings, business meetings, even shopping times are written there. Are all of these more important than romance? More important than your marriage? If they seem to be more important right now, later on you may find that your partner has been having an affair. It need not come to that, but it is important to get your priorities right. Mark off three hours every week or fortnight on your calendar for time together and do not allow anything to put it off. Make absolutely certain that the time is set.

CREATE A SPECIAL SPACE

It helps to make a special space for lovemaking to happen within. This can be in your bedroom or another area in your home. Before a date for lovemaking give the room a good cleaning—put shoes and clothes away and remove things that remind you of everyday concerns, such as newspapers, magazines, or toys. Place objects around the room that are pleasing to the senses—flowers, soft lights, or candles are wonderful. Burn incense and play music conducive to lovemaking.

Prepare not only the space and the time, but each other as well. Bathe each other's feet; massage and talk to each other. Massage puts you into the right frame of mind. If you are not confident about massage there are many good books and one-day courses where you can learn enough to be able to give a sensual massage. You might like to try this sensual massage sequence.

I know that many men reading this section on creating more intimacy through eye contact, talk, and romance will dismiss it or say they already know these things. But how many take three-hour sessions with their wives and actually do all of these things? Very few! Many men know these secrets, but doing it makes the difference.

Massage for the Senses

Make sure the room is warm and you are both comfortable. Ask your partner to lie on her belly. Rub your hands together to warm them. First pour warm oil sensually down her spine. Then place one hand at the base of the spine and one at the top of the spine and simply hold for one minute, while sending your love and compassion from your heart through your hands into your beloved. Proceed to massage the whole of the back.

Now, with your lips on either side of her spine, blow warm air from the base of the spine right up to the back of her neck. Do this a couple of times.

Kiss lightly around the back of her neck, around her ears. Nibble around her ears and the top of her shoulders.

Provide some firm massage around her hips and sacral area. This releases a lot of sexual energy. This is the area that acupuncturists work on to release and heal sexual energy. Using your thumbs, massage deeply into the sacral area.

Next, massage down the legs and to the feet, using long strokes up the inside of her legs and down the backs of her legs.

Ask her to turn over and massage the front of her body, leaving the genital area and breasts for last.

Kiss a point in the center of the chest between the breasts, in the heart chakra region, like a love kiss, for one minute or even more. Then kiss the groove of the left armpit and then the right armpit, one minute on each area.

Lie down or sit up and look into each other's eyes. Feel yourself becoming softer, vulnerable, and more open to love. Say affirmative things to each other, such as "What I like about you is . . ." or "What I appreciate about you is . . ." Read a poem that you have written for your beloved. Or read her some love poetry.

Creating romance is fun if you have the right attitude. As a child you often used your imagination in games to create special spaces for yourself and your playmates. I encourage you to bring that childhood playfulness into your lovemaking. You will find you are more imaginative and creative than you think, especially when you know the outcome is going to be sublime lovemaking. Try it just once and see what happens!

If you know you will never take the time to complete all the things I have suggested, then at least make sure the room is tidy, have some soft lighting, and play some music. Add something to the room that will distinguish this special session from your daily life.

Remember that you are a great lover. Anybody can be ordinary, but you have chosen to be an extraordinary lover.

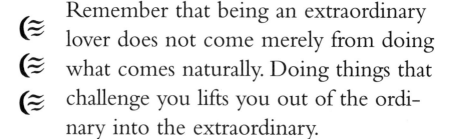 Remember that being an extraordinary lover does not come merely from doing what comes naturally. Doing things that challenge you lifts you out of the ordinary into the extraordinary.

4

Secrets for a
Healthy Relationship

Close, loving relationships provide the potential for the highest love-making possible. It is worth working on your relationship if you want to open up more possibilities in the area of your lovemaking, because as your relationship grows closer, your love grows deeper and sex gets better. There is nothing better than having a fabulous sexual experience with the person whom you love the most in life. Sex can be fabulous out of relationship, but it can be even more fabulous with a person who deeply loves and trusts you, because then you have the intimacy as well as the sexual passion.

The topic of relationships deserves a whole book, so I won't try to cover everything I have studied, experienced, and taught in this area. However I would like to point out some of the things that I feel have been a great asset in keeping my marriage together, as well as the relationships of many others with whom Diane and I have worked.

First of all, in discussing relationships it is important to point out that relationships in their current form in our society are not working. Statistics show that in Western societies more than 50 percent of all married couples get divorced. Once we fall in love we get married and take the vow to honor and love each other forever, in sickness and in health. Even though we may truly hope for this at the time, the evidence is that fairy-tale marriages, in which the couple gets married and lives happily ever after, are rare. Yet deep down many people still expect this to happen for them, and when it doesn't they feel deeply disappointed.

If, on the other hand, we had been conditioned to accept and honor "serial monogamy" as the norm, then we wouldn't put such pressure on ourselves or our partner to be happily married and in love for a lifetime.

But that is not how we are conditioned by the fairy tales and by society. Our society has decreed that we marry for love and that love should last for a lifetime. This is a wonderful proposition. However, because we are given little or no education on how to achieve it, it's destined to fail.

In *Challenge of the Heart* author John Welwood points out that "no earlier society has ever tried, much less succeeded at, joining together romantic love, sex, and marriage in a single institution." In traditional societies it was normal for marriages to be arranged by the families. Happiness was not the goal of marriage; marital union had more to do with family lineage and property. Feelings of love were never considered a reason for marriage; marriage for love was not considered until the nineteenth century. However it was regarded as degrading for a woman in Victorian times to have sexual feelings, so men often had sex with prostitutes.

It's important to understand the impact of this—to understand that you are a pioneer, one of the first of mankind to ever attempt to combine love, sex, and marriage. No wonder you have difficulties. It's not simply to do with you and your partner's inadequacies. It's a huge challenge and there is very little education on weaving together love, sexual passion, and marriage for a lifetime. That's why I love the work Diane and I do with couples on a journey into love. The average couple will not look at this type of education until they have big marital troubles.

What Diane and I teach is foreign to most people. As soon as we mention the work we do with love, sex, and relationships people say:

"We don't need it, but we know someone who does." Usually it is one of their friends who is having trouble with their marriage. What those people need is a counselor, therapist, or psychologist, not us. What Diane and I offer is education for happy couples who have chosen to explore the extraordinary in their love life and who are excited to learn all there is to know. They want to be great together.

When a man wants to be a great musician, singer, or engineer, he does not rely only on his own knowledge. He will seek the best sources of education available. The same is true for lovers who want the best. The emphasis on individualism in our society, on "doing your own thing," can work against marriage. Many couples who have gone off on their own personal growth paths separately from each other often find it difficult to integrate that individual growth in a supportive way in their marriage. I'm not suggesting that personal growth work should not be done. It is most important, but if you have done a lot of that it's time to create a balance between your individual needs and the needs of your relationship as a whole. Go to groups that support your loving relationship.

In our seminars with singles we find a lot more men and women are wanting to do that—to nurture and develop a long-term relationship and go on a journey into love and growth together. The AIDS epidemic accelerated this need. However, I believe that it is not only the fear of AIDS that has caused this to happen. I believe people genuinely are wanting to end the battle of the sexes and enter into a joint journey of personal growth and sexual, emotional, and spiritual fulfillment.

We are entering what you could call the "we generation," following the "me generation" of the past few decades. This is happening on a global level. We need all the education we can get to make our relationships work, so I hope you will try some of the secrets we share with you in this book.

GIVE YOUR RELATIONSHIP HIGH PRIORITY

Diane and I have decided to maintain sexual passion and a loving bond throughout our lives together, so we put a lot of time and energy and care into our relationship. We treat it as a very special entity. It is more important than each of our individual egos. It's something we work on as teammates, continually creating more and more love in our lives. It takes something more powerful than hoping, wishing, or desiring. It requires a lifetime commitment.

In the initial stages of most relationships, when men and women meet and fall in love, there is lots of love and energy and intimacy, lots of lovemaking and lots of passion. Then, after a period of time, many couples lose that passion. *The Hite Report* (1976) states that 85 percent of women claim that, after two years of being in a relationship or a marriage, they love their husbands but they are no longer "in love" with them. Some couples will say to Diane and me: "We still have sex, our passion still comes up occasionally, but it seems to have lost its sizzle, it's lost its juice. The intimacy and the opening that we used to feel in our hearts when we first met isn't really there anymore. We're not in love like we used to be."

There is a school of thought that believes this is natural, that this is what happens. Diane and I believe it is natural and it is what happens unless and until couples consciously choose to continue to create love and passion in their relationships. This is possible, but it requires a decision that this is something that you dearly want in your lives, something that you treasure, something that you believe will give you more from life than anything else.

Diane and I see the path of our relationship as one of the quickest paths to our own growth and our fulfillment physically, emotionally, spiritually, and sexually. We see our relationship as a vehicle through which we get a tangible experience of love. For this reason she and I have decided to put a lot of energy, care, and attention into it so that we experience more love in this lifetime. We know that at the end of our lives what will count more than anything else will be how much we loved.

Above everything else, we all want love. We can go through life and gain a lot of things materially and socially, but if we miss out on love then we will have missed the most important thing in life. The woman with whom you have chosen to live your life—your beloved—is the one you have allowed to get closest to you, and through her you have the potential to feel even more love in this lifetime. A lot of people make a common error. They put more energy into their careers, their families, or their chosen sports than into their relationships. They expect their relationships will progress satisfactorily while they get on with these seemingly much more important things. They do not realize that by supporting and nurturing the primary relationship they will be able to enhance and give more energy and creativity to all other pursuits.

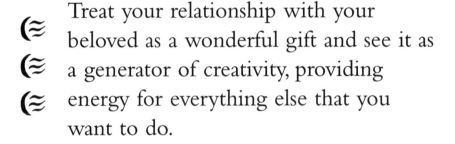

Treat your relationship with your beloved as a wonderful gift and see it as a generator of creativity, providing energy for everything else that you want to do.

Make an agreement to treat your relationship as high priority and put in the energy necessary to support that decision.

CREATING HARMONY WHEN YOU DON'T SEE EYE TO EYE

The truth is that no matter how much we want our relationships to run smoothly, disharmony still occurs. We get out of sync with our partners. We have disagreements, we argue, and sometimes we get angry and hurt and say things to our partners that we wouldn't say to our worst enemy.

What can we do about disharmony? First, we need to have the right attitude. If we have the attitude that conflict should not occur then we are always going to be under stress. Conflict is a part of growth and will occur in a healthy relationship. Very often the closer we get to our beloved the more conflicts arise, so as we confront uncomfortable situations together we need to develop the attitude that, although it can be painful, it is an opportunity to grow closer together.

Many people have the attitude that a good relationship must always be smooth and controlled, so they are unhappy and disappointed with marriage when it doesn't happen like that. They spend a lot of energy covering up the disharmony from others and they cover it up from each other until it gets out of control, and then the whole relationship explodes. So the first thing to have in your relationship is the understanding that disharmony is part of a healthy relationship, that it's natural. Loving couples strive for the joy of becoming closer and closer. They want union, but along with union comes dependence, which can make a man feel that he is allowing a woman to hold power over him. Men don't want to have to depend on women; to some men this dependence threatens their sense of masculinity and they resent it. Many women also resent feeling dependent on men, and this creates an ongoing struggle for power and independence.

That is why lovers will always go on fighting. The fight is simply a way to show each other they are still independent. We fight and feel like separating sometimes but it's not too long before we start wanting to make up, wanting to be held again, because the moment we start separating from our beloved we feel a need for the union. We miss the warmth, we miss the love, we miss the sex, we miss the feeling of union, we feel lonely and so do our partners. So we strive to create union again, and the struggle goes on. Part of us wants to be interdependent while the other part wants independence. It is important not to blame each other, because this is something that happens between male and female energies. Don't take it personally, and don't hurt the other for taking part in a significant element of the man–woman relationship game.

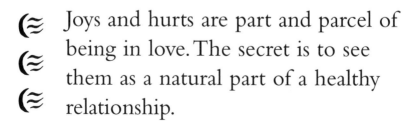

Joys and hurts are part and parcel of being in love. The secret is to see them as a natural part of a healthy relationship.

There is a well-known teaching that says: "In order to go forward you must first contract." The metaphor is that of a bow and arrow. In order for the arrow to move forward you must first pull back against the bow. This is like two people who pull away from each other, contract from each other as tension builds up, and then when it is released they move further forward in their relationship. A master archer knows to let go of the arrow as soon as the contraction is complete and his aim is taken. We need to become master archers in our relationships.

In the same way, if we are to move forward in our relationship we must learn to let go and not carry bad energy around with us for hours or days. Some of us hang onto our disagreements for weeks. We must learn to let them go, but how do we do this?

Shutting off and walking out of the room is basically saying: "Screw you!" and is an invitation for a huge fight. You must discuss the issue. If at some point you do head out of the room, make sure you come back open to talk. However, discussing your disagreement while you are in a high state of resentment can be very difficult and could perhaps lead to more disharmony.

Have you ever noticed when you start to discuss an issue how totally irrational your partner can appear? This is because women very often operate on feelings while men have been trained to operate on logic.

What should you do in these situations? The first step is to let go of having to be right and having to prove your partner wrong and move into the bonding process.

BONDING

Diane and I use a practice in our marriage called the Bonding Practice. Charles and Caroline Muir are excellent teachers of tantra, and many teachers of sexual loving instruct on similar exercises. Here is our version. It includes stopping the talking when you realize it's not going anywhere and agreeing to physically connect your bodies. Basically, as soon as you catch yourselves starting to pull away from each other, either physically by wanting to run out of the room or by closing down your hearts, one of you who wants harmony again asks the other to engage in the Bonding Practice.

It is important that you and your partner have agreed to do this in times of conflict. This process will help to keep sexual passion and a loving bond alive in your relationship. You should make a prior agreement to partake in the process always, so that when one of you asks this of the other you will agree to say "yes." It is not based on whether you want to, it is based on a decision you have made together in your relationship and that you both have agreed to honor no matter what.

If you find that you are so upset that you can't touch your partner, then have a shower or do whatever is necessary to get rid of that resistance and come back in ten minutes ready to do the practice. Never refuse to honor this agreement, because if you do you threaten the issue of trust in your relationship. Your partner has trusted you enough to drop the argument and ask for harmony. This is affirming that your relationship is more important than ego, more important than being right in this particular issue. Whatever you do, do not negate that trust by refusing to honor your agreement.

Suppose it is you who lets go first. You could say: "This is not getting us anywhere. I want to be in harmony with you. I want to practice bonding. We can discuss this later when we are not so upset. Let's put our bodies together." Your partner can readily agree or ask for some time, after which she must honor your request. The steps in the Bonding Practice are as follows.

THE BONDING PRACTICE

Step 1

Start in the nurturing position. Lie on your back while your partner lies beside you and rests her head on your chest. Place your right arm around your partner in a nurturing manner. She places her right hand on your heart chakra and you put your left hand on top of hers. Bend your right knee and place it between her legs,

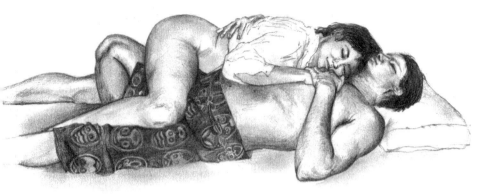

THE NURTURING POSITION

touching her sexual center. Her right leg is bent over yours so her knee touches your genital area.

This connects the heart center, where you can open to give and receive love again, with the sexual center, which, for a man, tends to open you more to wanting intimacy. For her, being held in the nurturing position tends to open her heart center, and touching her sexual center with your leg reverses her normal reactive behavior to close down sex to you in times of conflict.

Probably one of you will be resisting but, because you have an agreement to heal the disharmony, you will need to concentrate on letting go of any aggression, allowing the intellect and the emotions to become passive and taking your awareness to the physical body and breath. Sometimes it works to put on some soft, relaxing music.

Step 2

Now work with the breath to let go of any tension. If you are very upset you will find that you will be tensing your body and holding your breath, or you will feel your partner doing this. The secret is to reverse the process of shutting down to one of opening up. Breathe in with a long, deep breath through the nose and then sigh as you breathe out through the mouth—Aah! Repeat this at least ten times, coordinating your breaths if you can; otherwise make sure you are both doing deep breathing. Never allow just one of you to be doing it; both of you must participate.

As you breathe out, let go of any anger or resentments or the need to be right. Release all tension in the body, especially in the jaw, neck, and shoulders. As you continue with the breathing allow your mind to quiet, allow the inner chatter about the argument to be dismissed. Take your awareness instead to the contact points between your physical bodies, especially your heart centers. Focusing on the breath, consciously release all tension and argumentative thoughts until your body and mind are completely relaxed.

The requesting partner focuses on the heart being open—feeling love, compassion, caring, and forgiveness. Invite these qualities into your heart as a feeling or visualization, whichever works for you. Feel the warmth of your partner's hand on your heart center. Now focus on nurturing your partner like a child who has been hurt. Think of this as healing her inner child. Focus on that part of her that you really love beyond the part that has upset you.

Your beloved focuses on being nurtured and cared for and then shifts her attention to her hand on your heart, healing it and opening you more to love again. If it feels appropriate, she can move her hand from your heart center to your sexual center, gently cupping this area for a few minutes while you keep your hand on your heart center. This allows harmony between emotions and physical sexuality to develop once more.

You now exchange roles with your partner, gently repositioning before beginning. You need to spend at least five minutes in each role for this practice to be effective.

Step 3

Now turn to face each other and hold each other naturally, without your hands holding the heart or sexual chakras. Continue to breathe and let go, but do not say anything. Gaze gently into each other's eyes with love and compassion while tuning in to your own higher self, where having to be right or having to win the argument or having to change the other person is not important. What is important is to keep eye contact and be soft and vulnerable and see the part of your beloved that wants to be loved and wants to love. Act as healers for each other, showing compassion, care, and concern for your relationship.

Keep breathing gently. After a minute or so, or when appropriate, you say, "I'm sorry we were fighting. I love you." Your woman listens, breathes in, and internally accepts this. Then she says, "I'm sorry too, and I love you." Finish with a hug and a kiss.

It is most important not to say anything like, "I forgive you, but next time . . ." This would blow the whole process. You may as well not have done it in the first place. Do not talk about the issue, just hug and kiss and suggest a cup of tea or a walk. Maybe several hours later or the next day you can return and deal with the issue. Dealing with it immediately after the Bonding Practice is dangerous, because you are very open and sensitive when you have trusted enough to say "I'm sorry" in this way.

After you have completed this process you may not even need to discuss the issue again because you will find that the reestablished harmony and balance may well provide a new viewpoint, and whatever happened is no longer an issue for one or both of you. If you do discuss it, you may find you come up with other solutions to the problem that you might not have reached while in a reactive mode. It is always easy to feel that you are right and the other is at fault or not quite how you would like them to be or to behave.

In reality, neither of you is perfect. You both contributed to the disharmony in some way. By looking within and forgiving and by balancing the energies between you, very often circumstances begin to change.

In summary the three steps are:

1. Let go of the argument and ask to do the Bonding Practice.
2. Go into the nurturing position and practice deep breathing.
3. Face each other and forgive.

THE POWER OF SURRENDER

What you are doing in these three steps is surrendering your ego and honoring your true feelings to keep the sexual passion and a loving bond between you alive. In my relationship with Diane my ability to surrender is one of the most powerful qualities I possess. Surrender is not the same as compromise. Compromise is like saying, "Well, have it your way," but underneath that statement is the subtext, "but I'll get you later." Or you may concede because she wants you to, but you feel resentful, and that can build up over the years.

Surrender is not submission. Submission is being weak, where you give up and let your partner win the argument. Surrender is letting go totally and giving over to a truth higher than yourself. In this case the bonding of your relationship becomes the highest truth, not you winning the argument or allowing your beloved's wants and needs to be more important than your own. It is important to honor your truth, your needs, and your wants. Surrendering is a powerful stance.

The Bonding Practice is very potent and, in our experience, once the energy is balanced it is more likely that a solution will be found to whatever caused the disharmony in the first place.

USE THE BONDING PRACTICE
TO NURTURE EACH OTHER

You can also use this practice when you sense there is disharmony in your relationship and you can't define the cause of the problem. Instead of letting it brew and eventually boil over into something more serious, ask for or offer your partner a nurturing practice, depending on the situation.

Malcolm and Brenda, who attended one of our couples' workshops, said they found this the most beneficial of all the practices we gave them. Malcolm uses it whenever he sees Brenda getting uptight about work or the kids, from premenstrual tension, or for any other reason. Instead of trying to figure out just exactly what is wrong, he simply asks her if she would like some nurturing and they spend ten minutes in the nurturing position.

Malcolm explained: "We do it wherever we are in the house; usually on the sofa in the lounge room, fully clothed. We don't finish by saying, 'I'm sorry,' because there is nothing to be sorry about. We hug and I tell her I love her. The kids see us hugging a lot more and I think that's good for them too. What's more, Brenda doesn't appear to get as uptight with them after being nurtured."

Brenda said she likes to use this practice whenever she feels she is not getting the attention she would like from Malcolm. Malcolm works from home and sometimes spends hours in his office on weekends. "Sometimes I get angry because I feel he thinks his books are more important than me. I know he has deadlines to meet, but that doesn't help me. Now, whenever I feel like that, instead of getting angry I simply go into his office and say I'd like some nurturing. The beauty is, he has to agree to it immediately or in ten minutes' time. It works wonderfully for me."

Malcolm said that very often he gets so involved in his work that he is not aware Brenda wants his attention. He is grateful for her approach because he knows the disharmony that could eventuate if he worked all day without acknowledging her: "She would pay me back later by not giving me attention in bed!"

When Diane and I go away on our vacation seminars we make this a daily practice for couples. It takes only ten minutes so it is an excellent practice to use in your relationship, especially for busy couples who often say they do not have time for making love or they are too tired after work. You will notice that as you connect with your beloved every day for these ten-minute periods you will find the time to make love more often. Busy couples often do not touch each other in a loving way because they are too busy finding the time to do everything else! They might be great friends and have meaningful discussions, but their love-making becomes less and less frequent.

If you sometimes find yourself in this situation, talk about it and try the Bonding Practice every day for just ten minutes. I am sure you will have positive results. If your partner is not willing to try it then I suggest you need to take a close look at your relationship. If ten minutes a day is too much to ask then there is not much hope for a deeply loving relationship to develop. Yet this is why you came together in the first place.

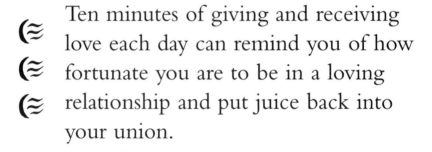

Ten minutes of giving and receiving love each day can remind you of how fortunate you are to be in a loving relationship and put juice back into your union.

POSITIVE COMMUNICATION

One of the common problems in marriage is that often each of us feels we are not being appreciated enough for what we do, yet this is often because we forget to voice our appreciation of our partners. Commonly, we do not realize that we get into the habit of finding what our partners do *wrong.* We need to make it a daily practice to scan all the things they do to find what they are doing *right,* and tell them how much we enjoy it. When was the last time you told your beloved that you really appreciate the meals she cooks? That you think she is doing a great job with the kids? That you really appreciate her organizing your social calendar? During the next couple of days, whenever she gives you a suggestion about something, say, "That's a great idea!" Even though you may not intend to take action on it, at least give her some acknowledgment for contributing the idea. Say, "That's a great idea, thanks for that, I'll consider it!" Or next time she does something that she perhaps does every day, such as preparing a meal, say to her, "I really appreciate your cooking dinner for the family."

So often a man takes it for granted that his partner knows he appreciates what she does. Women also often take it for granted that their men know that they are appreciated. Sometimes a woman won't say so because she's still angry about all the things he does that she doesn't like. Because she never acknowledges him, why should he acknowledge her? It grows into a competition for power, a battle. As teammates in love, men and women should be empowering each other to feel good, but instead they often get into the habit of fault finding and then they only empower each other to feel bad.

Diane and I enjoy watching couples at dinner. Often the husband will share something and immediately the wife will make a comment that negates what he said. For example, at a social gathering recently a friend was telling us how great he felt because he had just completed staining the outdoor furniture. His wife immediately commented: "Not bad after six months of saying you were going to do it!" She could easily have said: "I'm really pleased with how it looks. Michael did a great job." But instead she took the opportunity to criticize him. Her comment might have been designed to get back at him for playing golf on Saturdays instead of spending more time with her.

At other times we hear a man talk about himself and his business successes and his wife feels she is not being acknowledged for her part in the success. From the way he speaks it is as though he is responsible for it all and that her support of him in his day-to-day life has nothing to do with his success. She feels she is not being acknowledged. Try to acknowledge your partner for something every day, even if only to say "thank you" for the evening meal.

COMMUNICATING WHAT YOU DON'T LIKE

I have talked about the importance of telling your woman things you do like, but what about the things you don't like, things that annoy you? Are you supposed to just ignore them? You could, but that keeps your relationship on a shallow level, where you show only your light side. With friends and acquaintances you may be afraid that if you say something that might upset them then they won't like you anymore. That, to me, is a superficial relationship in which you cannot tell the truth for fear of losing that person's love.

It is a great gift to live with a person to whom you can show your dark side. Your beloved sees your angry self, your sad self, your depressed self, your bored self, your pissed-off self and still loves you (hopefully). You should be able to speak the truth to your beloved about what you do not like about her or what she does. You do not get to do that with everybody. You only get to do it with the person whom you love and trust. It is important that you have a safe way to say this because you are playing with fire.

THE WITHHOLD: TELLING THE TRUTH

This practice requires a lot of trust. It also requires that you truly want to know the truth and are mature enough to hear it and that your relationship is secure enough to encompass this truth.

Sit opposite each other and look into each other's eyes. You begin the communication with your beloved's name: "Diane, there's something I've withheld from you."

She simply says: "Okay, would you like to tell me?"

You reply: "Yes," and then you tell her whatever it is. This withhold is something that you have not said through the day or something you have not done through the day.

It can be something simple. For example: "Helen, there's something I've withheld from you."

"Okay, would you like to tell me?"

You reply: "Yes. This morning when I got out of bed and you were in the shower for twenty minutes and I couldn't see in the mirror to have my shave, it really annoyed me."

It is very important that your woman does not make some excuse for her behavior or want to argue but that she simply says, "Thank you."

The withhold does not always have to be something that she does that upsets or annoys you. You also may say affirmative things that you should have said sometime. For example: "Helen, when I saw you getting dressed on Saturday night for the movies, I thought your hair looked really beautiful."

She simply says, "Thank you."

It is imperative that when your partner hears something positive she says thank you in the same tone as when she hears something she does not like, because it is important for her to realize that this is not about her being right or wrong. The purpose of the withhold process is to allow the two of you to release any tension.

When you have finished she simply says, "Thank you." Then it's her turn and she follows the same procedure.

"Brian, there's something I've withheld from you."

You reply: "Okay, would you like to tell me?"

She says "Yes. When you bring the car home almost out of gas and I am going somewhere and I'm late, I really get pissed off at you."

You simply say, "Thank you."

"Brian, there's something I've withheld from you."

You reply: "'Okay, would you like to tell me?"

She says "Yes. I really appreciate the way you always have fun with the kids after work and play games with them."

You say, "Thank you."

She continues for about five minutes, after which time you hug and the practice is complete.

After you finish the process it's extremely important that you don't discuss any of the issues, especially the ones that aroused any sensitivity. If you carry on further discussion about them the process will lose its power. Forget it! The process is over. The other person may or may not choose to do something about the issues raised. For example, if you raised the issue about your being unable to see to shave, it is really your issue, not hers. She may or may not choose to do something about it next time the situation arises.

The purpose of the Withhold Practice is not to propel either of you to do something about the issue. Rather, it simply enables you both to diffuse energy so that there's more space for you to reach a deeper level of communication.

The only way you get to appreciate how powerful this process is is by actually doing it with your beloved. Like the Bonding Practice, the Withhold Practice works brilliantly in times of disharmony. There is nothing more vital than learning an appropriate and productive way to verbalize the anger, the pain, the frustration, the joy, the happiness of living with your partner.

THE SEXUAL WITHHOLD PRACTICE

This is an advanced withhold practice only for couples who are really committed to their relationship, who are deeply in love with each other, and who want their relationship to be extraordinary. The practice requires deep trust.

To see if you are ready for this practice read this example of a woman's list of "withholds" from her husband. It was taken at one of our workshops.

- "Brian, there's something I've withheld from you. When we make love and you ejaculate before I orgasm I really get pissed off with you."
- "Sometimes when we are making love you start pumping too hard and it hurts me and it turns me off."

- "When we make love and you stroke your fingers through my hair I really like that."
- "I hate it when you make love to me and you've been drinking and I can smell it on your breath."
- "I hate it when you come to bed and you just assume you can make love to me even though you haven't been talking to me most of the day, not in a nice way anyway."
- "I really love the way you kiss my breasts, it really turns me on."
- "I've never told you this before, but most of the time I'm faking my orgasm."

Before agreeing to do this practice imagine that these things were being said to you. Decide whether you would be able to handle them and what you might say in response. All you can say during the Sexual Withhold Practice is "thank you." If you go delving into the whole thing afterward your partner will never trust you enough later to tell you the truth. If this is too advanced, and it is for many couples, an alternative process is to spend five minutes listening to each other. One person talks for five minutes while the other just listens and says "thank you" at the end. Then the other partner has a turn at speaking.

This practice seems simple but it is very powerful. Often you are not heard when you express something to your partner because she jumps in and defends herself, or you do the same. Then it becomes a matter of winning as opposed to being heard, until eventually one submits or gives up. Great! Maybe you win the argument but then you wonder why she's not feeling sexy for the next week. Remember, you are playing with fire, especially if you say anything negative about her attractiveness. (Maybe leave those ones out!) It's up to you and depends on the level of your relationship.

Men are very often afraid to say anything in the area of sexuality. Many women don't say what they want in bed because they are afraid their man will react to it—and if it has anything to do with his self-image as a good lover, he most likely will. So what are you both to do?

Can you tell each other the truth? You can as long as you do it in a non-blaming way in which it's very safe, you trust each other, and you definitely keep agreements. For the practice to be successful the structure of withholds has to be quite tight, with definite agreements that should never be broken. Withholds are not designed to change the other person's behavior; only the person can do that. Withholds are designed to give both partners the opportunity to release tension and to create more time together and deepen their communication.

FOLLOWING THE PRACTICES AND AGREEMENTS EXACTLY

Damien and Janet had been married for three years when they started using the Withhold Practice. They shared some emotional times while doing it but they found that, once they completed the practice, they felt much closer and more trusting of each other. However, they only ever did a sexual withhold once and it ended up in such a huge fight they said they wished I had never introduced the process to them.

When I questioned them further they admitted that they hadn't followed the structure. They started discussing one particular issue because what Janet said was so charged that Damien couldn't let it pass; instead, he immediately started to defend himself. Within some sessions, after some withholds, they said "thank you," while after others they entered into a discussion and then returned to the withholds.

That is *not* the way to do it. If you are going to use this practice it's essential that you follow the structure. Through our workshops Diane and I have introduced this practice to hundreds of people and it works wonderfully, but it is like using Grandma's recipe—if you play with the ingredients it won't turn out the same and you will most likely be disappointed.

EXPLORE THE EXTRAORDINARY
IN YOUR LOVEMAKING

You can explore the extraordinary by varying the ways you make love. When I suggest varying the ways you make love many people assume I mean to vary the positions or the ways you can have intercourse or the places where you do it. However, I don't mean simply changing the positions, although it is enjoyable to do that. Changing the place where you make love is important, too. After you have been in a relationship for some time you often adopt one favorite position and make love in the same place. When your lovemaking becomes routine you don't bother to make love in the kitchen or living room anymore.

I have proposed many variations for lovemaking that might seem unusual at first. The intimacy exercises and practices are themselves ways of making love. The energic lovemaking in chapter 8 and the Jewel-Honoring Practice in chapter 10 are ways of making love. A person skilled in the art of lovemaking knows that the number of ways you can make love is unlimited.

Marie and Nathan had been married for one year. Marie told Diane that they had lived together for six months before they were married and had enjoyed a great sex life. Then, after one year of marriage, their relationship had lost its sizzle. "We seem to have fallen into the habit of having sex after we go out on Saturday night, and that's it! I almost regret getting married now. I loved sex before. We were always experimenting with new positions and ways of making love.

"Nathan was a great lover and still is, I guess, it's just that now we do the same old routine. There's a pattern to it—we start off kissing, then he goes to my breast, then he goes to my clitoris, then he enters and waits for me to orgasm most of the time or I put my hand to my clitoris to bring myself to orgasm. That's the only variation. Then he comes and we go to sleep. I love it and it works, but somehow it seems to have lost its magic for me."

Marie and Nathan's story is typical of so many couples, especially those who have been together for more than five years. They get into a pattern and sex isn't exciting anymore. They still like sex, but it lacks the passion and the energy it used to have when they first met. Sometimes the reason for this is that the pair hit on a good combination of actions that work and they keep going back to them because they don't require much thought. That is attractive to a lot of couples who are too burned-out from their hectic daily lives—from business, kids, financial pressures—to put any creativity into their lovemaking.

Many men feel threatened if they are asked to do something new. In our workshops when Diane and I suggest they try a particular style, they often retort: "I didn't do it; I just like to be spontaneous and natural in bed. I don't want to follow instructions." Unfortunately, their so-called spontaneous and natural lovemaking is pretty much the same each time. Later on they wonder why they find that their wives are not wanting to have sex as much as they used to or that they are having an affair to recapture the excitement, to rediscover lovemaking that is different and fresh.

A study was conducted in the United States where couples were videotaped making love. Twenty years later the same couples were again videotaped and there they were making love in almost exactly the same way. Just as an individual can become so easily set in his or her ways, so can a couple in their lovemaking.

You might know many ways of making love, but how often do you vary your lovemaking? That's the question. Knowing is one thing but acting on it is another. When I introduced this to Ken, one of our students, he said: "We've been married for ten years and there's only a certain number of positions you can try. Add a little oral sex to that and what else is there?" Ken has lovemaking mixed up with intercourse. In our workshops Diane and I teach at least a hundred different ways to improve lovemaking. Most couples have never taken the time to explore these.

Ask yourself these questions:

- Do you think the amount of love that you feel now is all that is possible? In other words, do you think the amount of love that you can feel is limited?
- Do you think your woman's orgasmic response is limited to what she experiences now?
- Did you know your woman has the potential to orgasm for up to an hour?
- Did you know that you can be multiorgasmic?
- Did you know that you can orgasm without ejaculation?
- If you know this, have you experienced it yet?
- Did you know that sexual energy and love are the highest transmitters of energy in your body?
- You may have explored all the positions in the physical aspects of sex, but how much have you researched and practiced the emotional, the psychological, and the spiritual aspects of lovemaking?
- How often do you literally burst into tears or deep joyful laughter with the joy you experience while making love?
- How often are you and your beloved totally out of control, where you no longer have thoughts and you experience mystical or spiritual awakening, a kind of bonding with the source of all creation?

In some relationships the physical aspects of sex can be great, but there may be very little real intimacy and deep sharing on all levels of your being. Sex is sometimes used by men as an excuse for intimacy. A woman says she wants more intimacy and her man thinks she means sex. The question to ask yourself is: "How much does your heart literally burn and pulsate with love for your beloved while you are making love?" (I did not ask about your lingam, I asked after your heart.)

All of this and much more is possible for you to explore. By opening new horizons and possibilities in lovemaking with every woman you fall in love with, and especially with the woman with whom you have chosen to share your life, you can become an extraordinary lover.

If you have reacted negatively or found yourself short-tempered with any of those questions it is probably because you are feeling threatened. That is a common response, but try to stay open to learning because it is possible to experience lovemaking as spiritual. Couples in our workshops have repeatedly described such experiences. These are people who are willing to be opened to new experiences and prepared to become teammates in love and to work together to explore just how much sexual passion and union they can feel together in this lifetime.

Regardless of what society or your friends think about this, your ultimate potential for lovemaking is unlimited. It is so extraordinary that it cannot be described. If your sex life has lost its sizzle and you have reached the stage where you are contemplating new partners, then it is probably because you have stopped exploring with your present partner. You might say, "Well, I want to explore but she doesn't," and that may be true on one level. Yet on another level her heart's true wish is a lifetime of love and sexual passion with you. You need to be an extraordinary lover and, with your love and your lovemaking secrets, heal her of whatever has caused her to close down her dream.

MAKE THE TIME AND PLAN FOR LOVE

I want to explain in more detail the importance of making the time and planning for love. It has added so much to my lovemaking with Diane and to the lovemaking of those to whom we have introduced it, especially busy couples.

Diane and I have been married since 1979. We have three children and a successful business, but we spend hours making love because we give our relationship number one priority. We know how much lovemaking supports our marriage so we organize our calendar to find the time.

Saying "I haven't got the time" really means that something else in your life is more important. Yet I promise that, when you are in your eighties, when your body does not work or look like it used to, when you get an erection only once a week and when you come you barely feel it, you will wish that you had spent more time loving and making love when you were younger.

Are you always too busy providing for the family to enjoy the ultimate act of intimacy? Do not miss it! Do not put it off! Do not come up with excuses! Find the time for this greatest of God's gifts—the ability to make love.

I suggest you plan a weekend away together at least six times a year. Don't go away to sightsee or shop or to try out the restaurants the place has to offer. Take your own food and wine and lock yourself in your room.

People often go away for a weekend and only make love at night as they normally do. Plan the weekend to try out the things you have read in this book. Perhaps Saturday could be her day to try the things she wants to and Sunday could be your day. Even planning and anticipating what you want to do will bring back the sizzle.

As I have mentioned earlier, there are a lot of resistances to planning sex and putting aside the time because this is not spontaneous or "natural." So very often sex takes low priority in everyday life because it is not the exciting, special happening it used to be in the early days. It is ironic that people spend so much time and energy preparing for other activities and occasions. They put these events on their calendars, organize their business and family around them, plan to wear their best clothes and go to the hairdressers, and yet they cannot find the time to make love. Surely lovemaking, which is potentially the most intimate event two human beings can share together, deserves the same amount of preparation and anticipation.

SAY YES TO SEX

This is an advanced practice and it is one of the greatest secrets for keeping a relationship in harmony and full of love and passion. The technique is: "Say yes to sex." Make love every day, whether you feel like it or not.

Many couples will permit themselves a sexual experience only when absolutely everything is correct. Everything has to be right. The man has to be in his woman's good books by behaving the way she expects him to. He has to be feeling sexy and things have to be going well in his business and family life—no stress, no tiredness, no headaches, no emotional turmoil. And then maybe, just maybe, he will make love. The problem is that very seldom is everything just right.

Eddie and Carol have three children: Heather (eight years old), Peter (seven), and Sam (ten months). Carol explained: "When we were first married we had a lot of sex with no fear of pregnancy—I was already pregnant—and we were hot for each other most of the time. Now with three kids all we want to do at the end of the day is sleep. We like sex and love each other, but we are lucky if we make love once a month."

Tom and Cathy had been living together for one year. Tom said: "When we first started living together we were like a couple of cats in heat. We made love in every room in that house. We would rip each other's clothes off in the kitchen, in the middle of making dinner. I'd lift her up on the kitchen counter and have yoni juice for my appetizer. I remember those days. Cathy would wrap her legs around me and I would carry her on my penis from the counter to the table, to the chairs, to the sofa, to the floor. They were such passionate times. We'd often end up eating dinner at midnight.

"Now after only one year she just doesn't want to anymore. I understand she's busy at work and gets tired. So do I, but I'm still hot for her. When we do make love it's just ordinary, as if she's just doing it because she has to. It makes me feel like some sort of sex-starved pain to her."

How many readers relate to this?

Another couple, June and Barry, had been married for three years when they started their own business together. After five years of running the business, often working twelve hours a day, they had little spare time together. When they did take time off they discussed their business. June remarked: "We still love each other and love sex when it does happen, but we just literally haven't got the time. When we take holidays we make love a lot. It's just that our business takes up all our time. Otherwise our sex life would be fine."

These are typical couples who, when they first get together, have lots of sex, but when circumstances change sex revolves around whether they feel sexy or not. So in those circumstances what do you do? I will share with you one of the greatest secrets to the success of my relationship with Diane. We have an agreement to connect every day, whether we feel like it or not. We do not wait for the right circumstances, right mood, and right everything else. Instead we go ahead and have a lovemaking experience anyway to bring us into harmony and to give us energy to change the mood we are in.

If your partner says, "I don't feel like sex!" or "I'm too tired!" make love and change the mood; make love and give each other energy. It is exactly what you need right then. Loving gives you energy; it does not take it away. What rubbish we allow our minds to get away with! How ridiculous to say: "I'm not in the mood to make love!" Making love can change your frame of mind. Use love as a healing force to give you exactly what you want. Similarly, a common excuse is: "I haven't got the time." But do you watch television for two hours before going to bed?

Often when a man avoids making love it's because he feels under pressure to perform and he does not have the energy for a performance. He just cannot be bothered doing all the foreplay required to get his partner to orgasm. Often a woman does not want to be under any pressure to come, either because she is too tired or too burned out from the day's work.

I want to outline a practice called Daily Devotion that will solve these excuses of the mind and lead you to more pleasure, energy, and harmony in your relationship. It involves the concept of surrender, which is one of the most beneficial practices you can do in a relationship. It involves a deep understanding of the importance of having lingam in yoni a lot of the time.

In the early part of a relationship there is plenty of passionate lovemaking. You have lingam in yoni a lot. Most people think it is because they are in harmony, have lots of energy, and feel good when they first meet that they make love a lot. This may be true, but the opposite is also true. The more time you have lingam in yoni the more opportunity there is for harmony.

It is a great secret to know that when you have lingam in yoni it can be a source of energy and vitality in your life. It readjusts a couple's moods and aligns their energy centers. It readjusts the psychic equilibrium of each partner's nervous system, generating more energy to deal with circumstances in the external world and to change the feelings in each person's internal world.

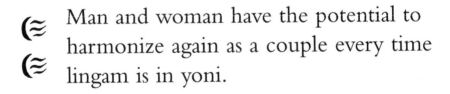

Man and woman have the potential to harmonize again as a couple every time lingam is in yoni.

Next time she says: "I don't want to make love because I'm not in the mood," you can reply: "Then let's make love to change the mood."

"I've got a headache!"

"Then let's make love to heal the headache."

"I'm too tired!"

"Then let's make love to give us energy."

"We are out of harmony, I'm not relating to you lately. We argue too much, how can we make love?"

"Well let's make love to heal that and harmonize with each other again."

Say yes to sex.

Remember, sex is an agreement. If one partner requests sexual loving, the other must say "yes" or give an alternative time. Never put it off a second time or you will create distrust in your relationship. In this case you each commit to treating your relationship as high priority. Let each other down on this one and you could be headed for an unfulfilling life together, or even for divorce.

INTRODUCING DAILY DEVOTION

Sex is a powerful agreement to make, but it is easy, very easy, if you follow this daily ritual that Diane and I practice. It is called Daily Devotion, and we have introduced it to hundreds of couples. We always get great feedback on how this technique has enhanced relationships. This practice is one of the best secrets I can share with busy couples.

I learned a similar practice from Dr. Stephen Chang, an internationally renowned expert on Taoist sexology. He calls this practice Morning and Evening Prayer. When it was first introduced to me it did not seem particularly powerful, but after practicing it for a week I changed my whole concept of what this technique can do. So don't treat it lightly. You may think you have done it before, but until you do it the way that we suggest for a period of time you won't appreciate its power.

This practice is a devotion to your intention to keep a loving bond and sexual passion alive in your relationship. You can call it Morning or Evening Meditation.

Of the hundreds of practices we teach this is the one from which we have had the most positive feedback. If you do not like to call it devotion or meditation or prayer, then simply see it as a harmonizing exercise, because that is exactly what it is.

In order to understand harmonization of male and female energies, let us first consider the basic natures of man and woman. In Genesis chapter 1 we read: "In the beginning God created Heaven and Earth." This conveys the polarization of infinity (God) into two complementary polar opposites represented in humanity as Adam and Eve. In the *I Ching*, the ancient Chinese book of divination and a source of Confucian and Taoist philosophy, man is represented by the yang (more active) element or Heaven's energy and woman is represented by the yin (more receptive) element or Earth's energy.

It is said that when these two complementary polar opposites are unified, harmony or tranquillity will be experienced.

To me this means that when men and women achieve harmony through unification of the complementary polar opposites they can have a tangible experience of God—an experience of the kingdom of Heaven, or the Divine, or a sense of oneness. This unifying principle is reflected in all religious symbols, which are representations of the spiritual purpose or meaning of the religion. By God I do not mean some supernatural personality in the sky; I am referring to the whole oneness embracing everything—endless universe, infinity, the Source, or any other name you may like to call it.

Man and woman represent the complementary polar opposites in humanity. Through intercourse they metaphorically unite Heaven and Earth's energies so the potential is there for a religious experience, a tangible experience of God. Couples remark that sometimes during lovemaking they seem to melt into each other and become one being. Some

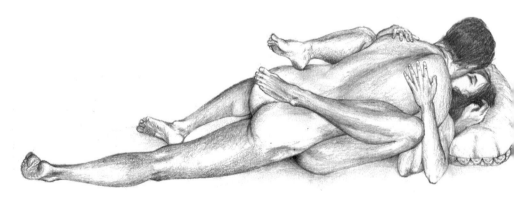

DAILY DEVOTION

describe the moment of orgasm as an experience of no thought. Eastern religions call this *samadhi,* which means "bliss" or "enlightenment."

As mentioned in chapter 1, some tantric and Taoist lovemaking practices (from ancient India and China, respectively) treat lovemaking as a meditation or prayer. If you practice meditation you'll understand that its purpose is the same as that of prayer—to increase your awareness and receptivity to God. It is a way of communicating with God, a way to experience oneness, peace, and harmony within your inner and outer worlds.

Daily Devotion is one of the best forms of meditation I know. I have no trouble practicing these meditations because I love sex, I love feeling my heart, and I love mystical experiences. Daily Devotion combines all of these. The practice itself is very simple, but do not be fooled by its simplicity; it is a deeply beneficial and fulfilling practice for you to incorporate into your relationship.

DAILY DEVOTION: THE PRACTICE

To perform Daily Devotion the woman lies on her back with her knees bent and wide apart. You lie between her legs in the missionary position. She then wraps her legs around your hips and locks her feet together, like a koala hanging onto a tree, with her arms wrapped around your neck. If this is not possible she can bend her knees and wrap her thighs around the outside of your thighs and place her lower legs between your legs, or whatever is most comfortable, as long as you are locked together.

You then put your lingam into her yoni or she places it in for you. Close your eyes and lock together with your mouths, legs, arms, and genitals. At first you may have just enough movement to maintain an erection, but then be still and enjoy the feeling of joy and gratitude that comes from being in union as one body with your beloved. Drink deeply of this experience, seize the moment, for nothing else matters but this precious time together. Keep your focus on the parts of your body that are connected and giving you pleasurable sensations. If your mind drifts, gently bring it back to where the genitals are connected and you are sharing each other's nectar. Think of it as drinking each other's juices—her yin essence benefiting you and your yang male essence benefiting her.

Daily Devotion presents a great opportunity for tremendous healing for your relationship. It will assist you and your partner to bond even more closely.

You can think of your love as a gift to the world or to your family or to your loved ones or to God. Start the day with Morning Devotion and conclude the day with Evening Devotion. During the devotion you are in a form of meditation and you can transcend time and space.

The devotion should last for at least five minutes, but even two minutes every day for one week will have a powerful effect. Do not be too concerned about the position, but do make sure the essences of the mouth and the yoni are being exchanged and your mind is continually brought back to your connection.

During this practice keep these thoughts in mind. "This is our devotion to our relationship, this is our prayer, this is our connection with our spiritual selves, with each other, and with God. Our prayer is for the blessing of our marriage to help heal each other of any disharmony that has occurred during the day, in our individual lives, and in our lives as a couple."

If the spiritual aspect of this practice does not fit easily with you, then forget it. Instead, use the practice as a physical, mental, and emotional harmonizing technique to bond your relationship closer together and to balance any disharmony that has happened between you throughout the day.

Daily Devotion can help you face any relationship disharmony and learn from it. See your committed partnership as an opportunity to learn more about yourselves. You learn nothing from running away and blaming your partner for her mistakes.

Your relationship can be a path to self-discovery. Through it you get the lessons you need to help you grow into a full, whole, and loving human being.

Divorce is our society's way of dealing with major discord, and this causes much heartache to a lot of people. It is sad that many people are prepared to go through the pain of divorce rather than confront the disharmony earlier in their relationships, before they irretrievably break down.

Daily Devotion is the opposite of running away from conflict. It involves coming close together, as close as physically possible for two human beings. As a daily ritual it can diffuse potential discord before it occurs. It is a far better solution than divorce.

Ben and Theresa are a typical business couple with three children. Ben runs his own printing business, requiring him to leave home at 7 A.M. each morning. They shared with us the effect that Daily Devotion has on their lives.

Ben said that very often he didn't arrive home until 6 P.M., feeling burned out after dealing with the pressure of meeting deadlines all day, every day. "When I got home I very often just didn't even feel like talking. Theresa would want to talk about the kids' problems and all sorts of things that I needed to do around the house and with the family. The kids wanted my attention also. It was too much, so I just shut off from Theresa and I'd go into my own space."

Theresa said, "When Ben was cold like that night after night I started to feel he didn't appreciate me anymore; not only that, but I started to doubt his love for me, too. Once we went to bed, if we did get around to making love he seemed to be too tired for foreplay and just seemed to want to get it over. He'd come, then he'd roll over and snore—and I wouldn't fall sleep. I was angry and I was frustrated. I'd finally get to sleep but it wouldn't seem long before the alarm rang. Ben wanted me to get up and get his breakfast."

Ben added, "Yes, yes I used to do that. But eventually I gave up expecting breakfast.

"'Get it yourself—I'm tired! I've got a headache!' was nearly always Theresa's response. So I'd grab anything that was quick to eat. I couldn't be bothered preparing a good breakfast. Then I would drive off and fight the traffic for half an hour and I'd always be pissed off by the time I got to work to start another bad day at the office.

"By the end of the week Theresa would be exploding over a matter I thought was insignificant. I would walk out of the house or turn up the TV or put my head in the newspaper, then she'd start drinking gin and taking pills for her headache. There was so much tension in our lives I was ready for a divorce, but I didn't want to face all the pain it would create and I was afraid that I wouldn't be able to continue to run a business without Theresa's support.

"Since you've introduced us to Daily Devotion I've experienced a complete change in my attitude, in my energy, and in my life. I can't believe it. It seemed too simple, but I have found it relaxes me at night. I don't have to gather up the energy to go through the whole lovemaking bit. I don't have to worry about bringing Theresa to orgasm. She said she loves just to be held and kissed every night because it makes her feel I love her and I'm not avoiding her or using her. She always sleeps restfully now and most mornings prepares me an excellent breakfast. I now go to the office feeling great.

"We always set the alarm five minutes early, and we've made it into a ritual to do the Morning Devotion as soon as we wake up. Frequently we are still half asleep, but it seems to fill me with energy by the time we are finished. I feel a lot better about myself and my relationship.

"My business dealings have become a lot less stressful. The same things are still happening but I'm handling everything better now, even the traffic. I've been a lot more interested in sex lately, and we've had some wonderful sessions after lying in Evening Devotion for five minutes for three nights in a row without doing anything else. By the end of the week, when we go into Morning Devotion, it usually turns into a fabulous lovemaking session. Before I was introduced to Morning and Evening Devotion, by the end of the week I dreaded going home. Now I can't wait! I honestly think this simple practice has saved our marriage."

Most couples report that Evening Devotion has the effect of relaxing them both before sleep, while Morning Devotion has the effect of charging them with energy before the day's work. It is ideal for busy couples. Everyone can take five minutes in the morning and five minutes in the evening, whether they are tired or not.

Ron and Lynette are another busy couple with great jobs and well-off financially, but after two years of marriage their sex life was disastrous. Lynette rarely had an orgasm, so there was pressure on Ron to try to get her to "come." She always felt this tension and was afraid she would not be able to—and so they would both end up disappointed.

After a year of failures and a lot of fights and blaming each other, he avoided her except when he became so horny he would make love for his own satisfaction. Normally he would watch television until very late so that he would be too tired to make love when he went to bed.

Some men do this! Ron didn't want to have sex with Lynette because of the disappointment it caused, so he avoided hugging and kissing her too. Too many men mistakenly believe that if they hug and kiss their partners in bed, they must also make love to them.

Lynette felt bad about not being able to orgasm, and whenever she saw Ron talking to other women she became very jealous, fearing she was losing the loving attention of the person she loved most. Ron later admitted that because he was not getting the sex he wanted, he was tempted to look elsewhere.

When they first came to our workshop Ron and Lynette told Diane and me that they had put sex on the back burner, rationalized that it was not important and that marriage was more about friendship. They had rarely had sex together during the preceding six months, so I do not know why they came to one of our overseas vacation seminars. I think perhaps they saw it as an opportunity for a much-needed break together on a tropical island.

Although they chose not to do a lot of the practices that Diane and I taught, they did try Morning Devotion, and it really worked for them. Lynette now gets the loving and attention she wants from Ron.

Lynette said, "I love it that we connect every day and yet there's no pressure on me to come. We know the devotion isn't about orgasm; we have time now to focus on our love and our bonding."

Ron said, "I love the fact that I've been inside Lynette two times a day. I didn't realize how much I was hurting her by avoiding sex. We think a whole lot more about sex now. I can't get it off my mind, actually. And instead of putting it last on our list of priorities it's now very important to us. We've read and talked a lot about sex, and we've discovered that, with the right healing, a woman's ability to orgasm can be increased dramatically. In fact, we found out that sex therapists are having a lot of success these days in this area."

Lynette began to follow Diane's program for women to become more orgasmic, and she managed to experience orgasm through the self-stimulation program.

Lynette said, "We are not rushing it, but we know our sex life can only get better with our new attitude. Meanwhile, we don't have to avoid sexual contact because we have Morning and Evening Devotion."

SOME COMMON CONCERNS
ABOUT DAILY DEVOTION

"I find it difficult to go along with the idea of having contact with my partner regularly whether I feel like it or not. What should I do?"

Try to understand that Daily Devotion is a means of bonding. Your relationship is more important than how you feel—feelings change. If your relationship is dependent on whether you feel good you are going to be disappointed a lot of the time. Daily Devotion is part of an agreement that a conscious, loving couple make to be in sexual contact regularly, as a way of healing and energizing each other and bonding more closely.

"I find it difficult to not move."

This is merely a matter of learning to break old habits. You do not have to move just because that's the way it's always done in the movies. Lovemaking need not always involve movement. It is worth mastering total stillness—a lot of women really love it!

"I tried Morning Devotion once and it did nothing for me."

This is because this kind of energy exchange is subtle. Many people do not appreciate it the first time because normally their sexual focus is to have a mind-blowing, ecstatic experience, and if it's not that it's no good. You need to refine your tastes to all aspects of lovemaking and appreciate the subtle as well as the ecstatic experiences, the same way you can refine your taste and appreciate a wider range of food. Do not give up after the first experience; you need to practice Daily Devotion for at least a week to appreciate its effects. Practice for a week without ejaculating and you will soon start to feel the energy.

"I'm not wet and it's difficult for my man to enter me."

Keep a lubricant near the bed. Use a water-soluble preparation, or simply use just enough saliva to get the head of the lingam in the yoni so that the juices can be exchanged.

"If I haven't got an erection, how can I do the devotion?"
You don't need to have an erection. Use some lubricant or saliva, then gently have your partner insert the head of your lingam into her yoni so that the essences are mixing. You will experience the same effect as when you are hard. When you are soft, the scissors position (see page 166) is a good way to keep the lingam from falling out of the yoni.

"After doing Daily Devotion for a week without ejaculating, I found I had an aching scrotum."
Then why don't you go ahead and have a great orgasm? Not during the Devotion practice but in another lovemaking session. If you are young and healthy there is nothing wrong with having an orgasm. If you are weak and healing your body, then you should reserve your orgasm and use the techniques described in chapter 7 to relieve the swollen prostate and pelvic congestion.

"I start off all right, but because we are not moving I lose my erection."
Don't worry about this. If you wish to stay erect, your partner can squeeze her yoni muscles or move a little to keep you stimulated.

"Does Morning Devotion always have to be man on top?"
No, although traditionally man's energy is the yang energy and woman's energy is the yin energy. Being on top charges a man's yang energy, while being on the bottom charges a woman's yin energy.

I suggest that if your sex drive has not been as strong as normal and you want to build up the strength of your erection, have your woman take the upper position in Morning Devotion. Take as much nourishment and joy as you can from feeling the warmth of her yoni, the weight of her breasts on your chest, and the shape of her hips on your tummy. Do not ejaculate during that week and I assure you that, at the end of that time, you will be as hard as a rock—full of love, appreciation, and passion for your woman.

A final point I want to make about Daily Devotions is that it is important in the early stages of practice, especially in the first month, not to turn the devotion into a full lovemaking session. What can happen is that your partner may not feel like making love one night but will allow you to enter because she honors your request for Evening Devotion. If you continue to a full lovemaking session you break her trust, and she may not allow you to enter her the next time you ask. It is so important that your woman knows she can trust you in this process. Of course, if she asks you to continue then it is fine to do so.

WHAT TOUCHES MY HEART

This final, simple practice works very effectively in our workshops. May I suggest you use it after the Bonding Practice or after the Withhold Practice—when you have released the charge and you want to feel connected again, but the relationship is still tender. Or you can use it as part of your weekend away.

Over dinner, say to your beloved: "What touches my heart about you is . . ."

If your partner does not know anything about this practice, just say, "I'd like to share with you what happens to my heart when I am with you. Would you be willing to hear that?"

Perhaps after she hears it she will share with you, too.

Any discomfort you feel about trying this exercise will quickly dissipate after you experience its effects. Do not dismiss it because it sounds so simple. Try it several times to get used to it and you will find it's very powerful. The practice is structured like this.

OPENING YOUR HEART

Start with the eye-gazing exercise. Look at each other and breathe together for five minutes, then shut your eyes. Place your hands on top of each other over your heart chakra. Breathe to your heart area to feel your chest open and start to see yourself as a loving, compassionate, and joyful person. Imagine yourself as that person in your inner world; allow a smile on your face.

After a minute or two, open your eyes while your partner keeps hers shut. Look at your partner and think of the times you have had together. If it is your beloved whom you have been with for some time, think that in front of you is the one who opens your heart the most and sometimes closes you down the most. She is a vehicle for you to feel more love in your life; she is a great gift.

Ask if you may stroke her hair and then gently stroke her hair and face. Next, ask her to open her eyes. Then say, "What touches my heart about you is . . ."

Each time you complete a statement your beloved breathes in, absorbing the affirming energy, and says, "Thank you."

One couple allowed me to tape what they were saying and permitted me to share it with you. This is what Collin said to Mary.

"What touches my heart about you is that you really enjoy having a drink with me when we get home from work. What touches my heart about you is the way you give me a hug during the day. What touches my heart about you is just living with you, the feel of you in my arms, your smooth skin. What touches my heart about you is your happy laugh, your beautiful eyes, and your fantastic legs. What touches my heart about you is how sexy you are."

This is what Mary said to Collin.

"Collin, what touches my heart about you is the way you look lovingly at me when I am getting dressed in the morning. What touches my heart about you is feeling your loving embrace while we're making love, and the way you rub my shoulders after I've had a hard day. What touches my heart about you is the way you try to do your best for me and the kids. What touches my heart about you is the way you cuddle into me when we wake up in the mornings and the way you tell me you love me more and more each year we are married."

This kind of spoken affirmation is simple, yet powerful. Often in relationship we don't feel that what we do is appreciated. When you practice this affirmation exercise regularly you make a moment to say those things that you appreciate about your partner; you get to feel empowered by each other. That is what a relationship should be about—teammates in this life, growing together, living together, experiencing as much love as you can together and as much joy as this lifetime has to offer.

WHY STRUCTURED PRACTICES?

In my twenty years of participating in teaching seminars, it is my experience that theory makes no difference unless it is put into practice.

Deep learning for me always comes from experience, not just theory. You can know all the theory that has ever been written about whole-body orgasm, but that is nothing compared to the experience.

Today in the better personal-growth seminars, theory is put into practice through the use of structured exercises. The structure makes it safe for you to be honest and assists you to deal with issues in a non-habitual way.

People don't realize they have developed clever ways to avoid encounters that move them into new areas, but in order to grow everyone needs to challenge themselves and to take risks that, by their very nature, can be uncomfortable at first because they are new.

Many people know theoretically that it is good to move out of their comfort zones, yet they cleverly avoid it. The structure of these exercises makes it difficult, if not impossible, to use the usual techniques of avoidance. An example of this is where the woman asks her partner to spend more time with her. They can discuss it, but if he provides enough reasons and "logical" excuses to make her feel wrong, she may give up. When this happens a real issue has been reduced to a chess game of clever conversation, and although the woman has given up on one level, she feels hurt and disempowered on another.

Structured communication exercises always leave both partners feeling empowered because each person gets an equal opportunity to speak her or his truth.

Try the structured exercises and practices in this book. In some I make it clear that you must not interfere with the "recipe" or you will not get the same cake; others can be played around with in your own way. The exercises act like a third party; they make sure that each person gets his or her say and is heard by his or her partner. Those with a rigid structure are potentially very powerful. They have been done hundreds of times and they are perfectly safe as long as you adhere to the structure.

5

Making Love as Long as You Choose

Sexually, men face two major difficulties throughout their lives. The first is as a young, virile teenager being unable to last long enough to satisfy a woman, or even satisfy yourself. After weeks of anticipation it is often all over in a few minutes. Do you remember those times? Or are you still in the position of sometimes not lasting as long as you would like? What an embarrassment it is for a man of any age to ejaculate too soon. Not a happy memory.

Not a happy memory for a married man either, especially if your wife does not want sex as much as you do. When she does, you ejaculate too soon and she is left feeling frustrated and sometimes angry. Even though she might not say so or show it, she feels it. Not good times for a man of any age. I would rate ejaculating before you want to high on any man's private list of embarrassing times.

Be honest about this. If it is a problem sometimes and you want to do something about it, the first step is to acknowledge it to yourself. Remember, you are not the only man who faces this difficulty.

The second major difficulty is that, at some stage in your later years, you will no longer come too soon—you won't come at all. You won't be able to get an erection or, if you do, it certainly won't stand up as straight and hard as it used to. Very often your woman's sexual energy has increased, because most women reach their sexual prime when they are over forty. There is the opportunity for sex but you can't do anything about it because your sexual energy is not as strong. If you do get an erection and ejaculate, instead of the mind-blowing explosion it used to be it barely trickles out. It's more like a squeak than a roar. If you haven't experienced this yet, I guarantee that at some stage it will happen.

However, there is something you can do about it, as this loss of function is not necessarily a part of aging. These major difficulties can be overcome through learning the essential techniques of ejaculation control.

I'd like to share with you two typical stories of men who participated in our workshops. One was Luke, eighteen, and the other was Rob, in his late fifties. This is Luke's story.

"When I was fifteen I was so sexually charged I didn't actually think about much else. Even the movement of the school bus gave me an erection. I'd be putting my books over it, worrying that I would still have it when I was getting off the bus. Later on, when I started meeting women, we would cuddle and carry on in the backseat of the car or wherever we were. By the time I touched her vagina I'd be so hot that I'd be too excited to enter, or if I did enter it would be all over too quickly. Sure enough it wouldn't be long before I became erect again, but the second time was never as good and the third time was even worse. I never told anyone this was happening, so it was a great relief to talk about it in Kerry's workshop, where I was first introduced to ejaculation-control techniques.

"I practiced the techniques by myself at first. It was great that there were practices that I could do without a woman, because I wasn't always in a relationship. Then I practiced with a girlfriend. It took some time but I persisted, and my girlfriend had her first orgasm. She admitted she had been pretending in the past, but this time she'd actually 'come' and it made me feel great."

Rob related this story.

"After I turned forty I noticed that my desire for sex wasn't as strong as it used to be. After I turned fifty my erections were certainly not as strong, and yet my wife's sexual energy was increasing. I found that I was staying away from home a lot of the time. I played more golf than ever before and came home late from work. I was either consciously or subconsciously afraid of not being able to fulfill her sexual needs.

"I noticed that after she turned forty she became an angry, nagging woman and we continually argued about all sorts of things. Now I see it was her frustration about not being sexually satisfied. I'm sure it was to do with that, because since I've learned these techniques and she is getting sexual satisfaction, she is much easier to live with. I'm retired now and we make love sometimes three times a day.

"I didn't realize there were so many men out there who are secretly unhappy because they aren't satisfying their women the way they used to. I also didn't realize there are so many frustrated women out there, so many angry women, not getting what they need, all because of the lack of education in the art of lovemaking. I wish I'd had more sexual education when I was young. In my youth I wasn't even aware that women had orgasms. I'm really glad that I have much more sexual knowledge now."

The stories Luke and Rob related are typical of many of the people with whom Diane and I have worked. With them we have shared many kinds of sexual secrets. Although the skill of ejaculation control is not all there is to lovemaking, it's vital to getting what you or your beloved want from making love. There is a prevailing view that skill isn't what lovemaking is all about. But if you don't have skill how can you experience something new? If you don't know how to peel an orange you will never taste the sweetness of the fruit. Without skill and control over your ejaculation you will never experience the pleasure that lovemaking has to offer.

Of the teachers I have met who are trained in these skills and of the students I have taught, each has expressed to me the deep satisfaction it gives them to be able to choose when to ejaculate and when not to. You might doubt that it is possible to make love as long as you like and at any stage in life. I too was skeptical when I was first introduced to this possibility, but my experience is that my erections now are just as strong as they were when I was eighteen. I can make love as many times in the day as I wish and feel energized after the lovemaking. When I do choose to ejaculate, not only is it as powerful as when I was eighteen but I also experience multiple orgasms. Even though I was extremely virile as a teenager, I never experienced that!

Any man with the desire and persistence to practice can develop himself this way, no matter what his age. Although different problems occur at different ages in life, the techniques achieve the same results—an experience of better lovemaking than you ever dreamed possible.

The strength of your erection and your ability to last as long as you want without ejaculation is not all that lovemaking is about. This skill alone does not guarantee you'll be a success in bed. The ability to feel love and intimacy and express these feelings with sensitivity and passion is also what being a good lover is about. Men who are able to feel their love and share these deep feelings will never have a shortage of women in their lives.

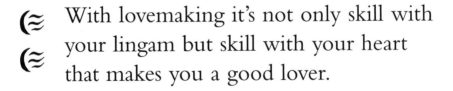 With lovemaking it's not only skill with your lingam but skill with your heart that makes you a good lover.

A lot of people use the term *making love* to describe the act of having sex, but to me making love is quite different. When you are not in a loving relationship and you are having sex purely for the physical pleasure it gives, I call that *sexing*. It doesn't mean that you don't care for, respect, and nurture each other, but it isn't the kind of love you can have for someone with whom you are in a deep relationship. Lovemaking to me is quite unique, a blending of your sexual passion—the heat in your genitals—with the deep love and intimacy you feel in your heart.

In a loving relationship it's a real awakening to conscientiously stop in the middle of lovemaking and ask yourself: "How much love am I feeling right now?" and to be aware throughout your lovemaking of how much love you are actually feeling, as opposed to how long you can last. Usually your mind is preoccupied with how much longer you can go before ejaculating. "I wish she'd come. I can't last much longer! God, it feels so good! Oh no, I'm coming. Oh damn, now it feels like she wants more and I'm finished!" Does this thought process sound familiar? It is for many men, and has been a common manner of preoccupation for the thousands with whom I have shared these secrets over the past twenty years.

I am personally indebted to my teachers for sharing these secrets with me, and I am grateful for the amount of freedom and feelings of self-worth, satisfaction, and deep joy they have given me and will continue to give me. I intend to be sexually active and vital in my nineties, not from positive thinking or willpower but from a deep understanding and practice of these secrets.

Most men who are open to learning about lovemaking realize that a woman's sexual energy takes longer to warm than a man's sexual energy. The Taoist Chinese tradition refers to a man's sexual energy as being that of fire, while woman's sexual energy is that of water. When fire and water get together the fire goes out, and this is what happens in lovemaking. If there's no education the fire goes out—the man ejaculates and the water is barely warmed. With skill, the man's fire can warm the woman's water through the techniques of ejaculation control. A man needs to be able to last long enough to warm the water to a state of climax to satisfy his woman.

THE IMPORTANCE OF
EJACULATION CONTROL

Techniques for ejaculation control are described in great detail in Taoist and tantric texts from ancient China and India, respectively, and, although the information is fantastic, it is often so complicated with detail and with Chinese terminology or Hindu methodology that it is difficult to read and understand.

Unless you have a background in Chinese medicine or have researched that particular culture, it is often quite difficult to put the techniques into practice. In my earlier studies I fell into the trap of getting so caught up in mastering the skills and understanding the philosophy that, even though I found myself becoming a great performer, there was something missing. The experience was often superficial and was more concerned with technique than loving. Diane especially felt this and reacted to it.

My intention is to keep techniques and terms as simple as I can so that the practice becomes more important than the understanding of terminology. However, for as simplified as I can make them I don't want to mislead you into believing that these lovemaking skills will work for you the first time you try them. As with learning any other skill, you need to practice each one before you can do it easily. In the early stages your mind might be focused on "getting it right," but once you master the practices, things flow, just like learning to dance. It's a mind and body skill, not just mental concentration or willpower.

Some of you will try these techniques and get immediate results, especially those of you who have some understanding of working with energy in your body through yoga, t'ai chi, massage, or dance. However, I have taught these techniques to hundreds of men with no background in these areas—and with great results. To master the skills takes some training. It's common sense that if you practice something regularly you will get better at it more quickly.

You have probably placed lovemaking high on the list of things you can enjoy, so it's worth spending the time to master these techniques.

The value will be enormous because sex is not a faddish activity. Lovemaking is something you'll be doing regularly throughout your life, whenever you are in a relationship. So the time you spend now developing these skills will benefit you for the rest of your life. As a man it will always make you feel good to know that during lovemaking you can let go with your pleasure, your joy, your excitement—any time the energy takes you—and still last as long as you want.

CONTROL—NOT TENSION

The word *control* often implies tension—fighting against something—but this is not the type of control I'm talking about developing. With these techniques I want to focus on working in a relaxed state, a manner of control like meditation. You can be in control in such a way that it's not a fight; rather, you're totally flowing with the energy—centered, experiencing everything that is happening. When you are learning to dance you are very much in control, and there's a certain rigidity to your movement because you concentrate closely on every step you make. Once you have mastered the steps, although you are in control you can move more freely to the music. It takes a lot of training to achieve the end result.

Some of that training can be done separate from lovemaking. A tennis player in training will practice certain strokes over and over again, then when he's playing a match he doesn't think about the strokes or the practice. Because of the training the stroke becomes automatic. If your partner wants to help you with the training while making love, then that is ideal. You become teammates in the game of love, with the goal being more pleasure for both of you. It's a good game to play!

Learning to be a good lover is essential, so that when you meet a woman with whom you want to form a relationship you will be far ahead of the lover who enters and literally blows it the first time. Single men spend a lot of time looking for the right woman. When and if you find her you'll need to have something special to offer her.

Having a good lover is incredibly important to most women.

Whether they admit it or not, every woman would love to have fabulous, orgasmic sex and feel loved. According to some research, some men ejaculate within three to five minutes of movement within a woman. You can't create a heightened sexual experience for her in three to five minutes! If you have the ability to be there with her totally as long as she wants, feeling the love instead of having to concentrate on facilitating orgasm or not coming too soon, she will think you're great.

> Ejaculation control will help create longer lovemaking sessions where you will be able to give and receive much more love. It will help you to reach a stage where there isn't any line between loving, touching, and actually making love.

This is what every woman wants, and you can achieve this when you master these techniques.

SECRET #1:
THE PC (PUBOCOCCYGEUS) MUSCLE

The first and most important thing to learn in mastering these lovemaking techniques is how to strengthen your pubococcygeus muscle, or the "love muscle." This is the major muscle of contraction in male and female orgasm. Strengthening the PC muscle helps to strengthen your erection and increase the sensations of your climax, which is very important in older years.

The PC muscle extends from the base of the spine, where it is connected to the tailbone (the coccyx), to the front of the body, where it is connected to the pubic bone. It is the PC muscle you use to cut off urination in midstream.

Just as you can tense and release your fist or tense and release your shoulders, you can tense and release the PC muscle. This will exercise the muscle involved in sexual pleasure.

Try it now to give yourself the idea of what I'm writing about here. Tense your fist and feel your biceps muscle tighten, then release—totally. Now see if you can tense and release the biceps muscle alone.

Muscle isolation practice will help you to isolate the PC muscle.

The next time you urinate, try to stop the flow in midstream to get a feeling of isolating and activating the PC muscle. At first you may need to tighten the whole pelvic floor, which includes the anus muscle and perhaps the lower abdominal muscles. Some men may need to tense the whole upper body to pull up the PC muscle.

See if you can locate the PC muscle. Flex it, even if your whole body tightens. Just as you isolated the muscle in the biceps from the fist, you can totally relax your upper body and still tense the pelvic floor.

Try it now as you are reading this. Your pelvic floor is tight but the rest of your body is relaxed. As you practice this regularly and your PC muscle gets stronger, you will be able to distinguish it from the nearby muscles. In the earlier stages do not concern yourself with this—just tighten and release all the muscles in this pelvic floor area, including the anus and buttocks. Continue to tighten and release several times.

Later, stand in front of a mirror and continually draw up and release this PC muscle, as if you are holding back urination. You will notice that you can make the penis move up and down as you tighten and release this muscle. If you can do this, then you know you are exercising the right muscle.

Now that you have located this muscle you can begin to strengthen it. Incorporate these simple exercises into your daily routine, independent of your lovemaking sessions. Then the exercises will become habitual and you won't have to set aside a special time to practice. For example, you can practice while you travel to and from work. No one will know what you are doing.

 Strengthening the PC muscle is one of the greatest sexual secrets a man can know.

You can strengthen this muscle with the following exercises.

PC HOLD

Contract the PC muscle as if you were holding back urination in midstream. Hold it and count to three, then release. Make sure the muscle completely relaxes before your next contraction. Hold it again, then release.

Draw it up now while you are reading this book. Hold, count to three, and release. Do this at least twenty times in your first session.

You can build up to whatever number of repetitions is comfortable for you. I suggest you commit yourself to five minutes on the way to work and five minutes while traveling home.

You can practice this exercise while you are sitting or standing, walking or resting. It may assist you if you combine it with the breath. Breathe in as you contract a muscle. Hold your breath and the contraction for a count of three, then make an extra strong contraction. Now release the muscle and the breath together. Do twenty cycles at a time. If after a week of practice you experience any soreness, take it easy. The pubococcygeus is like any other muscle—if you overdo it in the early stages, it can become tender.

FLUTTERING THE PC MUSCLE

Start this exercise by contracting the PC muscle. Tighten the muscle with a squeeze contraction, hold momentarily, then release completely. Squeeze, hold, and release while breathing normally. Concentrate on each contraction as you do it. The contractions are as strong as before, but they are made approximately one per second, like a heartbeat. As you get better try fluttering the muscle at approximately four contractions per second, and then much faster. I think of a butterfly's wings fluttering. You can feel the penis, the lingam, moving up and down. Complete three cycles of twenty contractions.

Incorporate these exercises into your daily routine, or do the one you find easier. Practice every day, with normal breathing. Make sure you relax the muscles between contractions—this is very important. Relaxing pelvic floor and buttock muscles during lovemaking is crucial to lasting longer. As the PC muscle gets stronger it's simple to gently spread the energy out of the genitals during intercourse, and the urgency to ejaculate passes.

Muscle-contraction and release practices to apply during intercourse are detailed in chapter 7.

Ancient Chinese emperors would have Taoist sages train their sons in these techniques. To test if the sage was proficient enough to teach the son, the sage would need to be able to place his penis in a glass of water and, using his PC muscle, sip the water through the penis until the glass was emptied. The more proficient teachers could do it with oil. Such a person would obviously have no trouble with ejaculation control.

I'm not suggesting that you try this, but it is important to understand the potential strength of the PC muscle in men. If your job involves sitting for long stretches of time without movement in the pelvic region, the muscles can become very weak over the years. People in these jobs are more susceptible to prostate trouble and may experience difficulty around the age of forty, and sometimes earlier. If you work in one of these jobs but have sex a lot, you will be getting some exercise in this muscle, because it's often only when we are making love that this area of the body gets exercised. So if you have a job that involves a lot of sitting, you may need to compensate by making love at least twice a day!

In the United States men participate in competitions where they actually attempt to lift different weights on their lingams.

One of my students, Brian, was nineteen when I met him. In exceptional physical condition, he was a young, healthy guy who enjoyed training and sport. When I introduced him to these techniques to strengthen his PC muscle he was amazed. He said he had just never thought of exercising that particular muscle.

Brian started to use the five-minute exercises I gave him, not once or twice a day for five minutes, as I had suggested, but for up to one or two hours a day at different times. He said that the muscle got very sore after one week so he had to rest for a couple of days. After that he made it part of his daily routine—five minutes each morning and each evening.

After one month's practice he became very proficient at this technique. He would play a game with his girlfriend, Sharon. He'd get out of the shower and start to romance her. When he got an erection, he'd say: "Watch this!" He'd stand back and drop his erection within ten seconds, then say: "I bet I can get it back up in ten seconds." He'd use his mind and his PC muscle to strengthen it, drop it, and raise it whenever he wished. Brian claimed: "It makes me feel good to run it instead of it running me. My mind is no longer in my penis."

Sharon told Diane and me what an amazing experience it was for her when Brian practiced these skills during lovemaking. "Brian had always been able to make love for a long time, but it was usually after he'd ejaculated the first time and then entered again. The normal pattern was that he'd always be really passionate and excited and loving toward me during foreplay, and when he entered he'd be passionate for five minutes until he ejaculated. Then we'd wait a few minutes and he'd enter again, but he was never as loving and as passionate the second time.

"I often felt that he was just continuing for me, that he wasn't with me anymore but was trying to make me come—which didn't work for me. It made it harder for me to keep my excitement up when I was thinking that Brian was continuing only for my benefit.

"Now that he's learned this technique I can feel his energy building up and peaking after about five minutes. Then he slows down a little, does his PC contractions, and we continue. The loving and the passionate energies continue to build. The more excited he gets the more excited I get, because I know he's really enjoying me.

"When I do come Brian usually comes with me, but one night he managed to hold throughout my contractions and continued slowly making love to me. Then I felt his huge rush of energy and throbbing as he was drawing back on this muscle and it activated my orgasm again. We continued to make love because he still hadn't lost his erection or his semen."

Everyone at the workshop seemed stunned. I knew it was threatening to some of the guys, so I pointed out to everyone that what Brian and Sharon were experiencing is a sensational blessing and we should not feel threatened by it. It can be quite a threat to a man to know another man may be better than he is in bed. This is natural, although no man would like to admit to such a thing. The male ego would never allow it, so when some of the men heard how well Brian was satisfying Sharon they got a little defensive. It is important to realize that these techniques are not designed to boost the male ego. They are about learning to get more out of lovemaking.

When some of the women heard how well Sharon was responding, how much she was enjoying herself with Brian, they worried that they were not good enough and that their guy would start looking for someone else. Or they felt a little threatened or disappointed that Brian and Sharon's experience was not happening for them. This is a normal reaction also.

A lot of people deal with this sort of reaction by closing down to any further learning; or they start to defend themselves by finding fault with what is being said. If you are aware that these types of reactions may come up for you, then try to pass through that, stay open, and look for something positive. For example, with Brian and Sharon's story the positive reaction would be to share in the joy of their experience. If Brian had said they had received a pay raise, had bought a new house, or had won a big football match, everyone would have cheered and been really excited instead of closing down and being silent.

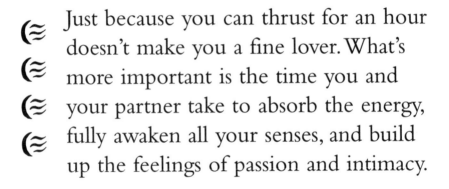

Just because you can thrust for an hour doesn't make you a fine lover. What's more important is the time you and your partner take to absorb the energy, fully awaken all your senses, and build up the feelings of passion and intimacy.

LEARNING TO RECEIVE

You need to be careful during lovemaking that you are not just performing to get a result. Men often find themselves doing that because they have been conditioned by a society that pushes for results or by parents who gave rewards only for winning, for getting a result.

Most men live their lives like this, until they become aware that they are so busy performing and producing results that they have forgotten how to receive love and nurture themselves.

In lovemaking men forget to receive the gift of love and healing energy their partners are giving. Men are often so busy trying to get a result that they miss the experience. Not too long ago women complained that men only used them for their own satisfaction. This may have been true for previous generations, but for aware men today this isn't the case.

Magazines and other media have put men under so much pressure to produce—to be good lovers, to nurture their women, to bring their women to orgasm—that now they are very often in the position of being unfulfilled themselves in their lovemaking.

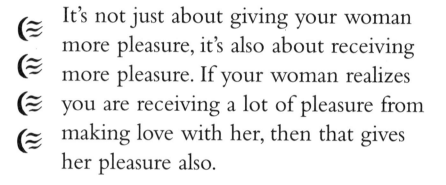 It's not just about giving your woman more pleasure, it's also about receiving more pleasure. If your woman realizes you are receiving a lot of pleasure from making love with her, then that gives her pleasure also.

This is what I understood was happening for Brian and Sharon. It was great that they were open enough to share their experience. If more people shared their lovemaking experiences we would learn and grow so much more as individuals, as a culture, and as a human race. However, the way we have been conditioned by society is that lovemaking is secretive, taboo, and private. Most of us find it easy to talk about our day at work, the weather, the latest movie, and our personal problems, but not about making love.

Doesn't it seem silly that we all know and respect the importance of love and yet we do not share with others the joy of our lovemaking experiences? Lovemaking is potentially a time when we can feel the most love in our lives, but we don't talk about that. I'm not suggesting that you immediately rush out and discuss such things with your friends. However, once you feel they are as well educated sexually as you are, it is a healthy thing to do.

SECRET #2: BREATH CONTROL

What most men do as excitement builds up and they get close to climax is move harder and faster and breathe heavier and faster, or else they hold the breath.

If we are to reverse the flow of sexual energy, the best way to do it is to breathe slowly and deeply and rhythmically. Even if you do move rapidly and your partner is moving fast too, keep your breaths long, deep, and consistent. Breathing does not have to match your movements. As you breathe in, imagine breathing in all the love essences, the scent, the beautiful sensations, and the images of your lover's body. Drink deeply of every magical moment of your lovemaking; do not miss one minute of this experience.

Here is a helpful exercise you can practice separate from lovemaking. It's an excellent meditation for single men to practice. This exercise is an advanced technique of breath and PC-muscle control, using the PC-strengthening technique discussed and practiced earlier.

COORDINATION OF BREATH AND THE PC MUSCLE

You should preferably sit in a chair for this exercise. Imagine the opening of your penis is like a straw. Engage the PC muscle and "sip" energy up through your penis the way you would sip liquid through a straw. Make a soft sipping sound to assist you as you practice.

Imagine that nectar is being drawn up through your penis, right up the spine to the base of your neck, right up to the top of your head. Now lock that energy in by pulling your chin into your chest and stretching the back of your neck. With your back straight, hold the energy for a few seconds. Then release the chin and the breath while making the sound "aahhh." Bear down on the PC muscle and release it as you let the breath go.

Repeat the exercise as many times as you can.

It is important that you actually feel the energy rise and fall, and not just visualize it. This process can last for a period of five minutes. It's a good idea to try out this practice on your morning erections to test if you really can do it and that it's not just your imagination. See how many contractions it takes for you to make your penis go soft.

If you practice yoga you may prefer to sit in the cross-legged position. Yogis often do this exercise with their legs crossed so that one heel presses on the PC area. Some people do it sitting on a tennis ball or something similar that presses on the PC area.

If you feel a little dizzy afterward (because you are actually drawing energy up into your head), then try taking the energy up only as high as the throat; swallow; then breathe out as you feel the energy going down again.

Rub your belly strongly after the exercise, eighty-one times clockwise and eighty-one times counterclockwise, to spread the energy through your body. If you continue to experience dizziness during the exercise, then contract the PC muscle as you breathe in and out but do not sip the energy up to the crown. As you release the PC muscle and breathe out, feel the energy spread throughout your body.

(Similar exercises are done by women to assist in childbirth—for them it's important not to take the energy to the head, but simply to squeeze and release the PC muscle.) Coordination of the PC muscle and breath is excellent training for lovemaking, the kind of lovemaking where you have control over your ejaculation.

SECRET #3: MUSCLE TENSION RELEASE

The muscles of a man's body are conditioned to respond in a certain way as he builds toward ejaculation. They help him to ejaculate quickly. How did this happen? It's certainly not what a man wants to happen when he is with a woman!

These muscles probably were conditioned at puberty. Young boys like the sensation of ejaculation and so they masturbate like crazy to get that feeling as quickly as possible. As they begin courting girls, sex is often in limited supply, so when they get the chance they go for it. Very often there is a lot of tension when adolescent lovemaking doesn't happen in a safe and private place. Afraid that someone will see them, teenagers try to get it over quickly.

When I was about eighteen my brother, who was away on holidays, gave me the key to his house. My girlfriend and I had had sex only in the car, so my heart was pounding a thousand beats to the minute before we even got into bed. I had just entered her when lights started flashing, sirens blared, and the house was surrounded by police. The neighbors knew my brother was on holiday, saw and heard noises, and called the police. You can imagine how I felt—tense, frustrated, nervous, guilty—and I didn't even get to climax. Eventually everything was explained and we went back to bed. I wasted no time. I quickly entered, peaked, and the pressure and tension were relieved. Unfortunately for my girlfriend it was all over in a few seconds.

These urgent energies, these types of experiences, this pushing to orgasm to get the sensation, this secrecy, this pressure to go fast gets caught up in male bodies and their response mechanisms.

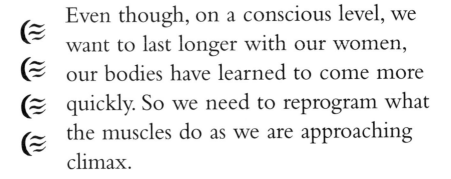

Even though, on a conscious level, we want to last longer with our women, our bodies have learned to come more quickly. So we need to reprogram what the muscles do as we are approaching climax.

We need to learn how to relax the muscles as they begin to tense. The subconscious mind is also conditioned to climax quickly because sex is often associated with secrecy and guilt. Subconsciously it's best to get it over swiftly because we don't want to feel guilty for too long. Even if as sexually educated men we may know it's necessary for our women's pleasure for us to last longer, our bodies, our muscular systems, and our subconscious minds already have been programmed to climax quickly. The subconscious is more powerful than the conscious mind.

Do you know what happens with your body's responses and your thoughts as you are nearing climax? Because your body is conditioned to climax quickly, the muscle necessary to cause this will automatically start to contract. Your breath will do what is necessary to assist you in climaxing quickly. Your mind will become stressed and your thoughts frantic as you fight the urge, especially when you know your woman would like to go much longer.

However, if you can observe your conditioned response you can also work at reversing the conditioning. It's not difficult—it's just a matter of awareness and a little training. Biofeedback works on the same principle. If, for example, you are suffering from stress, you can be linked to biofeedback machines and learn to find trigger points to release certain muscles before they tense any further. It works very effectively.

I'm not suggesting you link yourself up to biofeedback machines while making love. Could you imagine going into a clinic and saying, "Hi, I've come in to practice a little ejaculation control, so just link me up to one of those machines and I'll go ahead. You watch the machine." You don't need a machine to learn these techniques. You can teach yourself!

The best way to do it is while masturbating. Think of it as a self-pleasuring experiment to derive some invaluable feedback on yourself. If you are a single person and masturbate regularly, this self-pleasuring experiment won't be any problem for you. However, I know that many men in steady sexual relationships will not have masturbated for years, and you may experience resistance.

While studying at More University in Berkeley, California, I was given a similar exercise in a sensuality and sexuality course. I had a strong resistance to masturbating. I was married and felt I was past that now; I didn't need to do it anymore. However, it was explained to me that it wasn't masturbation but a self-pleasuring experiment to learn about myself. With some encouragement from Diane I went ahead and I learned enough to take a major leap in ejaculation control, not only through the strength of the PC muscle, but also through relaxation.

THE SELF-PLEASURING EXPERIMENT

Find a safe, private space and lock the door. Use a lubricant if you wish. Pleasure yourself for at least twenty minutes and, each time you approach climax, just before the point of no return firmly hold the head of your penis with a closed fist with no movement until the energy subsides. Keep the hand in place until your erection starts to soften a little, then continue to stroke and approach climax again.

Repeat this cycle several times. You can complete to ejaculation and climax if you wish after you have tried it at least five times; however, climax is not the point of the exercise. The point is to note what is happening as you approach orgasm.

What is happening with your breathing as you are getting close to climax? Are you holding your breath? Are you panting? What muscles are tensing? Are you tensing your shoulders, your face muscles, and (more importantly) your buttocks, your pelvic floor muscles, and the genital region? What's happening in your mind? Any tendency to get there quickly? Any fighting of the pleasurable feelings? The goal of this exercise is to start reversing some of this conditioning. This can be done through the use of the breath, thought release, and muscle relaxation.

What to Do with the Breath

Slow your breathing to long, steady breaths. Basically, breathe the opposite way to the way you normally do to achieve climax quickly. If you breathe through the mouth, try to breathe through the nose. The idea is to cool down, not heat up. That doesn't mean you fight your feelings, the enjoyment and excitement of orgasm. Indeed, you try to enjoy them more.

What to Do with the Thoughts

Thought release is another helpful technique. As you feel your mind rushing toward climax, slow down your thoughts. Try to delight in the subtle energies of mild arousal, the pleasurable feelings that occur long before the highly excited phase. Drink deeply of the sensations at this time and stop and breathe the sensations through your entire body. Imagine them spreading everywhere, not just in your lingam.

When you are getting close to climax, use your mind to relax your muscles. If you are tensing and fighting your mind, stop all movement, breathe deeply, and as you release your breath spread the energy and absorb the amount of pleasure. Breathe deeply with each breath and spread the pleasure.

Most men ejaculate when they can't take any more pleasure. What you need to do is to increase your pleasure threshold. This can be accomplished by taking yourself to peak but not climaxing on the first surge. Repeat this process and, as the energy builds up around the genital region, breathe deeply, hold the breath, and then spread the energy on the out-breath. Imagine the energy moving through your limbs, through your fingers, through your toes, relaxing your entire body and releasing all your tight muscles.

What to Do with the Muscles

As the energy builds up and you feel your muscles tighten, consciously relax them. Especially be aware of the buttock muscles and the pelvic floor muscles.

If you haven't had any practice releasing muscles, do this simple exercise. Lie down on the floor and work through the muscle groups in your body. Begin with your feet or your hands. Tense those muscles only, then relax. Move slowly through each part of the body. Try tensing and relaxing your shoulder muscles as you read this page; release your jaw muscles by dropping your jaw.

Men carry so much tension around with them, yet they often are unaware of it. You can combine the thoughts and breath to release tension—breathe in to the tense muscle, hold while the muscle contracts, then release the muscle and the breath together while making the sound "aahhh." Thoughts, muscles, and breath release are wonderful techniques to use to prolong your lovemaking.

The techniques related to the breath, thoughts, and muscles can be practiced alone or during intercourse, but I recommend that you initially practice them separately so that later, during intercourse, you won't have to concentrate on technique. They will occur naturally. If your lover is happy to work with you in the development of your lovemaking techniques, then that is a great gift.

MALE VIRILITY DRUGS

Viagra—and all the potency drugs that will follow—are powerful ingredients in sexual relationships, improving things for some but causing lots of problems for others. This is especially the case in a situation where a man's revitalized potency is not welcomed by his partner and he starts looking for other women to test himself on.

These drugs are not chemically designed to increase desire, but for many men, once they start getting erections again their desire for sex increases because they know they can perform. Performance, as you know and many women will tell you, isn't all women want from lovemaking; it is not the secret to making a woman love you. The drug doesn't necessarily help you make love longer. Although you may stay hard after ejaculation, the passion and intimacy have gone.

For some men these drugs may pose a health risk. In addition to the potential side effects, the ancient Chinese believed that as a man's life-force diminishes, so does his ability to get an erection. This is the body's natural protective mechanism to save him from overejaculating and los-ing more energy. By chemically inducing an erection most men then force themselves to ejaculate, even though they may not feel like it. The Taoists say this puts a tremendous strain on the whole body and affects health and life expectancy.

If impotence has been a long-term problem for you, and it is deeply embedded in your psyche that you need the drug for medical or psy-chological reasons, then my suggestion is to use it in moderation. Try natural methods first; the practices in this chapter do work over time. In the meantime, reduce the intake of the drug and increase the many other ways of satisfying a woman you'll have learned from reading this book.

6

Beyond Normal Orgasm for Men

Most men think they orgasm when they ejaculate. However, ejaculation is only one form of orgasm, and it is small stuff compared to whole-body orgasm. Whole-body orgasm rarely happens with normal ejaculation.

To understand this it is necessary to understand the chakra system. Just as we have physical organs in the body that perform certain functions, we also have energy centers that perform certain functions energetically for us. These energy centers are called *chakras.*

Traditionally it is thought that there are seven of these centers. The chakras are symbolic representations of the glandular, or endocrine, system within the body. Dr. Stephen Chang's theory is that a state of weakness or susceptibility to disease arises when one system—or in this case one gland—is deprived of energy for some reason. Not only is our task to reestablish the balance of the energy flow to overcome this weakness; it is also to raise the level of energy within the body to its maximum. Balancing and raising the energy to its proper level through the seven gland system is the Taoists' way of strengthening the immune system.

THE SEVEN CHAKRAS

Briefly, the seven chakras and their related glands and functions are identified here. (Please note that the location of the chakras varies slightly among different philosophies.)

1st chakra: Sexual glands (testes [male] and ovaries [female]; function is sexual energy; this chakra is often called the base chakra.

2nd chakra: Adrenal glands; function is balancing fluids in the body, including sexual fluids; this chakra is often called the sexual chakra. (Note that sexual functioning is shared between the first and second chakras.)

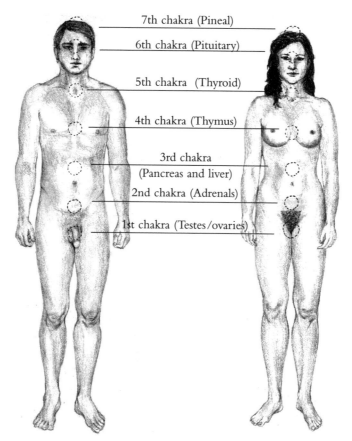

7th chakra (Pineal)

6th chakra (Pituitary)

5th chakra (Thyroid)

4th chakra (Thymus)

3rd chakra
(Pancreas and liver)

2nd chakra (Adrenals)

1st chakra (Testes/ovaries)

THE SEVEN CHAKRAS AND THEIR RELATED ENDOCRINE GLANDS

3rd chakra: Pancreas and liver; function is to maintain control of digestion and blood-sugar levels; this chakra is often called the power center.

4th chakra: Thymus gland; governs heart and circulatory system; this chakra is often called the heart center.

5th chakra: Thyroid gland; maintains metabolism of cells, governs growth; this chakra is often called the communication center.

6th chakra: Pituitary gland; governs memory, wisdom, intelligence, thought; this chakra is often called the intuitive center or third eye.

7th chakra: Pineal gland; affects other glands through its secretion; this chakra is often called the crown chakra and is associated with communication on a spiritual level.

> Most men when they ejaculate only experience a second-chakra orgasm. The energy builds up in the genitals until it reaches a peak, then the man has to ejaculate to release the energy. The experience is a throbbing of energy in the area of the second chakra only.

Occasionally, when that energy is very powerful, it will spread upward through the body, and the whole body starts to vibrate. When you consciously do this, building up the energy to such a state that it is actually being distributed through all the other chakras, then when you have an orgasm each of the chakras bursts. You experience a "seven-chakra orgasm," a whole-body orgasm.

At this stage the whole body feels like the penis. You may have experienced whole-body orgasm on many occasions but did not understand how it happened or how to repeat the experience. There are different ways to activate a whole-body orgasm. One way is through pleasure sessions where your partner looks after you and you surrender to the pleasure.

PLEASURE SESSIONS

In our workshops Diane and I often suggest that couples make time for a special pleasuring session in which the man is asked to lie back and totally receive while his woman strokes his lingam. He is not to reach out to hold her, kiss her, or touch her breasts or yoni, but is just to surrender to pleasure and not do anything but receive. This can be quite difficult for a man because so many men are into doing things, into production. When we are not performing, not producing results, not doing something, many of us have trouble just being. For example, how many of us, when relaxing on the beach, have trouble just being and instead feel the need to be doing something?

While participating in one of our workshops, Nicholas said he had not realized how much he was conditioned by the need to produce. When he stopped doing he had real trouble getting any pleasure. He said his penis went limp during this pleasuring process, and he did not feel like orgasming even after he had been stroked constantly for twenty minutes. He said that if he had been pumping for only five minutes he would have climaxed. He was amazed at how much his pleasure centered around his wife's response as opposed to the pleasure he was receiving. He only had to see his wife touching herself in front of him and he would sometimes climax within a few minutes of entering, without stimulation or any stroking. Yet he had been stroked for twenty minutes consistently and did not peak.

I told Nicholas this often happens to men when they are first learning to receive pleasure and to nourish themselves more. I also pointed out to him how amazing it is that, although the lingam has the most nerve endings of any organ in the body, after constant stroking for twenty minutes he did not peak. Yet if he watched his wife pleasuring herself in front of him, when he entered her he would not be able to last for even a few minutes—and the nerve endings would hardly have been touched. This demonstrates how much lovemaking is in the mind.

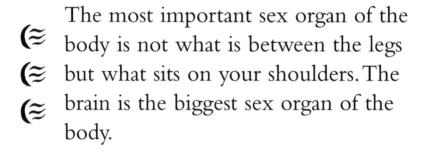
The most important sex organ of the body is not what is between the legs but what sits on your shoulders. The brain is the biggest sex organ of the body.

A woman enjoys pleasuring her man; she loves being in control of her man's pleasure. A man must realize that his partner deserves to experience the giving of intense sexual pleasure, too.

If you love her, then allow her this experience. If your woman offers to pleasure you, remember to acknowledge her and tell her how much you are enjoying it. In our workshop with couples Diane and I often incorporate a night of extended pleasure for the woman and another night for the man. This creates an opportunity to learn how to give and receive totally. Some of us give better than we receive, while some receive better than they give. Which do you think you do best? On these nights people get to experience both roles, because deep satisfaction from lovemaking should not be just one-sided. You are missing a great deal of pleasure if your only pleasure comes from giving.

Usually men are unaware of this. As Nicholas experienced, when men are put in this position of totally surrendering to pleasure they often discover how difficult it is for them. When this first happened to me I was staggered by the difficulty I had receiving and by how much my pleasure was determined by Diane's pleasure. If your partner wishes to give you a night of pleasure you will have your own experience of surrendering. You may, however, experience a resistance to pleasure.

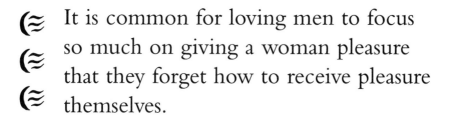 It is common for loving men to focus so much on giving a woman pleasure that they forget how to receive pleasure themselves.

RESISTANCE TO PLEASURE

Our resistance to pleasure is interesting. Most people would say they have no resistance at all, yet everyone has some resistance to pleasure. It is important to become aware of this and to work through it if you want to enjoy your lovemaking to the fullest. Let's take an honest look at this issue.

We live in a pain-oriented society. Listen to people talk, listen to *yourself* think or talk, and you will see that you often concentrate more on the things that are going wrong in your life—you focus on the problems rather than on the joys. It's a habit that we've fallen into. Read the newspapers. They are full of stories about adversity and pain. Why do you think they print more about the negative than the positive? It's because people are attracted to and fascinated by the dark side of life.

People will say, "Give me pleasure rather than pain anytime," or "We haven't the time to make love because we are too busy." Yet how many of us will sit down for two hours and watch television, seeing and hearing about the pain in other people's lives, instead of making love for two hours, which is about experiencing pleasure?

I wonder what is really happening? I suggest that there is a lot of resistance to intimacy in people's lives—resistance to love, to sex, to pleasure. It is important to understand these patterns in our lives and to consciously learn to increase our pleasure threshold.

Surrendering is a luxurious way to do this. A common resistance for men is fear of losing control. If a man can control the amount of pleasure he receives, fine, but if he is out of control, that is another issue. A man's pleasure often comes from being in control of his partner's pleasure rather than from being able to receive pleasure directly to nourish himself.

When your partner gives you one of these pleasure sessions you may want to take control. You might find yourself reaching out to hold her or kiss her or to touch her breasts, but the idea is to do nothing but totally surrender—lie back, relax, and be totally passive. Tell yourself you deserve this pleasure. Try to absorb it like a sponge, soaking up the energy of the gift of pleasure. If you can surrender totally to receiving then I promise you that the experience will provide a breakthrough for both of you on many levels.

WHOLE-BODY ORGASM

The greatest pleasures in lovemaking have happened to me when I've been able to give up control. The experience of whole-body orgasm is something you will never forget. I suggest you allow your partner to pleasure you manually for about half an hour, bringing you to a point of climax at least ten times before allowing you to ejaculate. This should put you into a high enough state to open up the possibility of whole-body orgasm, or at least give you an orgasm that will be more intense and stronger and last longer than a normal ejaculation. Instead of six to nine contractions you may experience fifteen to twenty, especially if you have not ejaculated for a week or so.

At first you will need to communicate this to her. You will also need to show her how to hold, by firmly encircling her hand around the head of the lingam until the energy levels out. Then your partner can continue to stroke you until you reach another peak. She then holds again, and repeats this several times. This proccess is called "peaking."

Communication is very important. For example, if she is stroking you softly and you would like it to be harder or faster, there is a right and a wrong way to ask for what you want. Instead of saying, "I don't like it that way, do it harder," try saying, "I'm really enjoying you giving me pleasure. Would you move a little faster and harder please?" You have acknowledged rather than criticized her effort. When she does as you request, say, "Thank you." If it is still not hard enough, don't say, "That's not hard enough. You don't know how to do it." Simply say, "That's nice, I am really enjoying it and would you go even faster, please?" Show her you are enjoying what she is doing.

(≈
(≈
(≈
(≈
(≈
(≈

Two things that will assist you during your pleasure session are riding the peaks and breathing correctly. The best way to ride with the energy instead of climaxing at the first peak is to make sure your partner learns your responses before climax. With familiarity, she will learn when to stop stroking and when to hold.

You might think it is silly having this communication structure, but in a loving situation it really hurts a woman when you say something to her that is a put-down. It is essential to support each other and be affirmative in your lovemaking, as you are teammates creating more love for each other. Don't be wishy-washy and nondecisive and say "Just do what you like." Communicate what you want. Then she will get what she wants, too, which is the joy of being able to give you this much pleasure.

And breathing is possibly the most important secret I can share with you to help create a whole-body orgasm. Breathing assists you in going through the resistances, in riding the peaks, and in spreading the energy through your entire body.

When reaching the peaks many men hold the breath and then tighten the muscles, especially the buttocks and the pelvic floor. Throughout this experience try deep breathing, as it helps break through any tensing pattern that may happen for you just before climax. It helps you to relax, it increases the supply of oxygen to the brain, and it reduces anxiety. You might like to try continual deep breathing—deep inhalation and exhalation—where you take in energy on the in-breath and let it out on the out-breath, continuing this in a cycle throughout the experience. It helps shift you from your thoughts into your senses.

Have your partner remind you continually to keep breathing deeply throughout the process while she does the cyclic breathing herself.

Continual deep breathing can create quite an awesome, whole-body experience. As you practice you will get better at surrendering, at riding the peaks and at using deep breathing, and you will find that you get higher and higher between these peaks until you have an experience of one continuous peak. You won't know if you have ejaculated or not because your whole body will be vibrating. At that point you will truly understand that ejaculation is small stuff compared to whole-body orgasm.

This process of peaking and breathing to create a whole-body orgasm can be practiced during normal intercourse, but the experience usually is not as powerful because you are not in a space of total surrender. Each time you come close to climax during intercourse use the techniques of the PC muscle pump, the muscle release, and the thought release so that the energy levels out. When you start to move again the energy rises, then you reach a plateau and then the energy rises again, spreading throughout the entire body. Eventually the energy builds up to such a degree that when you ejaculate it is so powerful that it shoots through all the chakras and you experience a whole-body orgasm.

Gary, who participated in one of our workshops, had an amazing experience with a woman who was trained in these techniques. Gary said: "I met Helen at a party and we made an immediate connection. We danced most of the night, then we went back to her place. After passionate kissing and undressing we got into bed and I took a condom out of my wallet and asked Helen if she would mind putting it on for me. Helen said: 'You won't need that.' When she said that I freaked because of AIDS. She added: 'I want you to receive pleasure, I want to look after you. I know what I'm doing and I ask you to let me do it.'

"It shocked me at first, but I decided I would go along with it. She laid me down and proceeded to stroke my entire body gently and teasingly. Every time I went to reach for her or hold her, she put my hand down and said, 'Just receive.' After being told this several times I got the message and surrendered to the pleasure.

"Eventually she reached my penis and she started to stroke it in amazing ways. I don't know what techniques she used but every time I reached the point of climax she would hold the head of my penis and the energy would rush through my body. Then she would start to stroke again. She seemed to know exactly the point at which to stop. She did this about seven times. I lost count but eventually something happened and my whole body started to go into spasm. My head thrust back and I didn't know what was happening. I thought I had ejaculated but I could still feel her hand on my penis so I had to ask her if I had. When she said I hadn't, I said: 'I don't believe it, I must have, I felt it. My whole body was in ejaculation mode.'

"She continued stroking and eventually I think I may have ejaculated, yet my whole body felt like my penis. It was the first time I had felt such an awesome loss of control. I entered into a space of total bliss. When making love before I had always been in control.

This was a situation where I was totally out of control and I experienced a whole-body orgasm. I decided I wanted to learn more about this. Helen told me about her studies and that's why I'm here. I want to learn more about the pleasure I can experience."

INJACULATION

Injaculation is a very old practice, one that I first learned from Dr. Stephen Chang. I was privileged to meet Dr. Chang in San Francisco in 1985. Dr. Chang is an internationally known scholar whose grandmother was a master physician. Her father was personal physician to both Empress Tse-Shi and the first Chinese ambassador to the United Kingdom. Dr. Chang has been trained in both Chinese and Western medicine; in addition to his medical degree, he holds doctorate degrees in philosophy and theology. He also holds two law degrees. He lectures worldwide on various aspects of Taoism and is the author of many books.

Dr. Chang shared with me some of the greatest sexual secrets that I now practice in my life. In return for this gift I brought him to Australia in 1988 for a lecture and workshop series in Melbourne. The energy and vitality he transmitted during those lectures was that of a young man. He was in his sixties then, yet he had the energy of a thirty-year-old. He taught me a great deal, including the following information.

During normal ejaculation the prostate enlarges with secretions to a stage where it can't contain anymore tension. Then a rapid series of contractions brings about ejaculation and the prostate shrinks to its normal size. As the prostate pumps it draws sperm from the seminal vessel. The secretions carrying the sperm then pass through the urethra and out the penis. If the PC muscle is very strong, when it is contracted it puts enough pressure on the channel that passes the base of the prostate gland to prevent semen from passing through. The body readily recycles the preserved seminal ingredients, transporting these juices via the lymphatic ducts into the bloodstream. This nourishes the body because, instead of the energy leaving the body as it does with normal ejaculation, it is reabsorbed, energizing the whole system.

The prostate itself needs to pump harder and longer to empty, intensifying the sensation so much that it can feel like five minutes instead of a couple of minutes. During normal ejaculation the prostate pumps between five and twenty-one times, but sometimes, as the area gets weaker, you may feel only one or two weak contractions. Whatever your sensations are now, let me assure you your experience will be greatly enhanced through learning the techniques of injaculation.

Some of our workshop participants have asked if it is feasible to use this method as a form of contraception. If a small amount of clear fluid containing semen escapes during injaculation it is unlikely to cause conception because, under normal circumstances, the penis shoots millions of sperm high into the vaginal canal for conception to take place. However, I cannot definitively recommend injaculation as a birth-control method because I used it in that way for years and then my daughter Lisa was conceived. If your partner is healthy and fertile, do not risk using this method. However, if the birth-control pill is causing side effects, you could combine this technique with other contraceptive methods.

Mastering injaculation is very difficult. It takes a healthy body, a strong PC muscle, and a lot of practice. "So what's the use of it to me?" you might ask. Fortunately there is another way you can experience injaculation without developing the PC muscle. This information is worth a million dollars.

INJACULATION EXERCISE

To create injaculation yourself you need to locate the perineum, halfway between the anus and the scrotum. When this point is pressed prior to the anticipated ejaculation and the ejaculation is stopped, the energy moves up into the body, through the meridians (the body's energy lines), instead of out of the body, as it does during normal ejaculation. Just before you are ready to ejaculate, reach around behind your buttocks and locate the perineum. Press it hard enough that the semen is not able to travel out of the prostate and through to the urethra. The pressure should not be too heavy or too light. If you press too close to the scrotum the semen will enter the bladder and be lost when you urinate. If you press too close to the anus ejaculation will not be stopped. The pressure must close the channels right at the base of the prostate gland.

You still feel the pleasurable sensations, which come from pumping the prostate, however no semen passes through the penis. The prostate has to pump much harder and longer to send the energy up instead of out, so the sensations are much stronger than they would normally be.

You might try this on yourself first, and use three fingers just to be safe. Your woman can press this point for you but it takes practice to locate the exact point. If the semen has gone into the bladder you will notice that the urine is bubbly and cloudy. In normal ejaculation, about one-third of the semen goes into the bladder anyway, so don't be concerned.

Again, anyone who has prostate or nonspecific urinary tract problems should not use this technique. I am not sure of the long-term effects of injaculation, but my advice is to use this only occasionally. I have a sense that it may put a lot of pressure on the lower area of the body if it is done too regularly. It is a great experience for a beginner, but once you learn the more advanced techniques you will find little need for this particular practice. You may use it when you want to feel the sensation of ejaculation, but reserve your energy for the next day or for another lovemaking session immediately afterward. It is an effective way to experience a whole-body orgasm because the energy is shooting up through all the chakras instead of down and out through the lower chakra.

VALLEY ORGASM

This is a more subtle, refined form of orgasm and it is one of my favorites. It is not so much a technique as an awareness and an appreciation of a more subtle energy permeating the body during lovemaking. The focus of awareness is not on the physical activity, nor is it on the climax; it is more on experiencing the energetic flow. The whole body orgasmic experiences achieved through peaking and injaculation can be likened to an overwhelming torrent of intense pleasure rushing through the entire body in waves, creating a peak experience of excitement. The valley orgasm is more like being bathed in gentle streams of subtle energies flowing through your entire body, filling each chakra with warmth and vitality, creating a sense of deep valleys of relaxation rather than a high peak of excitement. This does not diminish the experience, but if your mind has not been trained to appreciate subtle energies you might feel that nothing is happening and miss the experience, because you are always comparing it with the peaks.

A teacher once told me: "Your life will become twice as enriched if you can appreciate the pauses, the times in life when it slows down, when you've got nothing to do next. It would be very valuable and enriching if you could simply be with those moments and appreciate the stillness, instead of always thinking about what is going to happen next." As children we are conditioned by our parents to be expectant because they continually provide something for us to do and do not encourage us to appreciate the times when there is nothing to do, so often we don't know how to relax in the pauses. The mind says we are bored because we are unable to appreciate the "valley."

We have been conditioned by society to appreciate the active, the dynamic, as opposed to the subtle, the simple.

In our lovemaking we often miss the subtle energetics that are present because we are too busy focusing on the excitement, the movement, or the goal. To appreciate valley orgasm you need to train your mind to *be with the experience*, to be with the simplicity of what is happening in the pauses. An appreciation of the pleasure of a valley orgasm can be achieved through practicing methods that involve no movement.

Karezza is a practice that involves little or no movement. *Karezza* is an Italian word meaning "caress." It first appeared in English usage in 1883 in the book *Karezza: Ethics of Marriage* by Dr. Alice Brunker Stockham. The practice involves no movement and the couple stay in union for an hour. The mood is tender and loving. Only if the erection slackens do you move. The emphasis is on lovingly connecting and exchanging energy, rather than on genital orgasm.

It is important that your lovemaking session is long enough for you to feel the subtleness of the energy. Ideally it should last one hour, but in the early stages I suggest you try a practice for fifteen minutes, then gradually increase to one hour.

I read about this technique when I was fifteen, but I was never game to try it because I thought that the girl I was with would expect me to be moving. This is something that you need to discuss with your lover to understand the benefits of lying together.

If you have heard of this method and tried it, then try it again now with your new knowledge of ejaculation control. If you have not tried it, this is an excellent way to start experiencing valley orgasm.

A similar method to karezza is an Arabic practice that was developed out of necessity. A man needed a method of lovemaking by which he could satisfy an entire harem of women. By using this form of lovemaking with minimal movement, the man did not reach ejaculation; thus he could satisfy many women in one night.

BIOELECTRIC INTERCOURSE

Rudolf von Urban, M.D., whose book *Sex Perfection and Marital Happiness* was published in 1949, devised his own approach to making maximum use of subtle sexual energies. Von Urban reported that health problems such as high blood pressure, skin problems, and apathy were totally cured in some patients after a couple of weeks of bioelectric sex. He also reported that the technique was found to be extraordinarily relaxing. Von Urban reported that "some experienced renewal of their marriages, those who were in love became even more so and some long-term relationships which had been full of discontent suddenly enjoyed peace."

In brief, von Urban's theory was that the cells of the male body and brain and the female body and brain are opposites in terms of electrical charge. After prolonged contact of the skin, especially between moist areas of the body—that is, the genitals—the bioelectric quality of the skin changes. This change attracts the unique bioenergy in the cells of both genders to the surface of the skin, where they can be exchanged, resulting in benefits and perhaps ecstatic experiences. Scientists today have confirmed the electromagnetic character of the human skin, but have not yet confirmed the male and female electric cell polarities about which von Urban wrote.

Whether the theory is correct or not is immaterial. It is the practice of von Urban's method that matters. Von Urban gave easy-to-follow instructions that we paraphrase here.

MAKING LOVE WITH ENERGY

Shower or bathe and then, while completely naked, cuddle, kiss, or otherwise turn each other on. Lie in the scissors position (see the illustration on page 166). With the man on his left side, with or without an erection, place your penis just inside the outer lips of the vagina. Lie in this position for at least thirty minutes, focusing intensely on any genital feelings. Keep attention on the exchange of male and female polarizing energies taking place in the genitals. After the thirty minutes are up, have regular intercourse with genital thrusting, but stay in the scissors position. This should also last for thirty minutes. Male ejaculation is to be avoided. Should male ejaculation occur, the couple stays genitally fused for thirty minutes more from that point. This is to ensure that bioelectrical interchange between the lovers is completed.

KABBASAH

Sexual Energy Ecstasy authors David and Ellen Ramsdale, with whom Diane and I spent some time in California, describe another method of energy exchange that involves little or no movement. Called *kabbasah,* the only movement it allows is the woman's voluntary internal movement of her vaginal muscles. This skill is also known as *pompour.* In the Middle East long ago a woman who had mastered pompour was known as a *kabbazar,* or "holder."

In pompour the lingam can be fondled, caressed, gripped, massaged, milked, and rippled as a whole or in sections. During this style of love-making the man is totally relaxed. Neither he nor his woman moves the hips at all; all the action is internal. Each time the man feels as if he is losing his erection his partner uses pompour. This session should last a minimum of forty-five minutes to have a chance to feel the valley.

With training, women can develop the art of moving the vaginal muscles in amazing ways. Once you have experienced this with a woman who knows the art of pompour you will never forget it. The technique was most likely developed by the more talented sacred prostitutes in India and China and the geisha in Japan. Today men and women know little of this secret. The only time men experience anything like this is during a woman's orgasm, when the woman's yoni muscles involuntarily grip and contractions occur. If you know how amazing that feels, then that is just the beginning of what you can feel once your partner has mastered the art of pompour.

You can try any combinations of the above styles to give you an experience of the valley. What works well for Diane and me and I would like you to try is to first build up your love and sexual energy through kissing and caressing. Then you sit in a chair with your woman astride you. Move and make love in whatever way turns you on until you reach a peak of excitement, then stop—no movement. Relax in a loving embrace and feel the energy spreading—this is the valley. You do not have to do anything, just relax and feel the energy moving throughout your body. Only when the man or woman feels the energy has spread and the erection is going to be lost is a little movement and excitement required; then again relax.

You are not trying to build the energy up from peak to peak, to higher and higher excitement levels, as you were in the peaking technique for developing whole-body orgasm. Instead you are relaxing into the beauty of the valley, not going anywhere, just feeling the subtle waves of the valley. The idea is to prolong this deep embrace for at least an hour with no ejaculation. Eventually each chakra is bathed in the energy and you feel nourished on every level of your being.

Remember that during the pauses if there is ever a loss of erection the woman can use pompour; however, she must decide whether this is something she wishes to develop. Do not criticize her for not being able to use pompour the first time she tries it. Isolating and strengthening any muscle in your body is a skill that does not happen overnight.

Whichever way you attain it, through the valley orgasm you revitalize each other; you become regenerated through each other; you feel full of energy, more vital, more alive, and more radiant; and the ecstasy can last for hours and sometimes even days.

Each of these methods to promote valley orgasm involves periods of passive sexual intercourse, being still for at least half an hour or more, waiting for the electricity between the male and female energies to build up. It is in these periods of no movement that the valley can occur. After long periods of no movement it is common to experience sudden involuntary whole-body movements that feel like an electric current moving through you in waves of orgasmic sensation. I believe this is because during nonmovement the bioelectrical energy builds up to higher levels than normal.

What happens in conventional orgasm is that, because the excitement is built up and released quickly, it prematurely discharges the energy that, if allowed to build up slowly, could catapult the lovers into a state of involuntary movement. The only involuntary movement in conventional orgasm is at the point of ejaculation, and it is short-lived.

However, in the valley orgasm the involuntary movement can happen several times, sometimes continuously, sometimes at intervals of one or two minutes. You will experience a rush of energy shooting through your body and your muscles will involuntarily contract. But most often you experience a subtle wave of energy and warmth passing through you. It takes some practice to be able to be inside your lover without moving and to integrate higher states of sexual energy, because men are conditioned to move to gain pleasure. It is worth trying these methods several times to give yourself the opportunity to experience a valley orgasm.

In one of our workshops we introduced soft styles of lovemaking. I asked Allan and Annette to practice this nonmovement form of connecting every night for one week and then to report their experiences to us. Allan reported that when he first tried it he thought it was nonsense and a waste of time. He did not feel anything except frustration at not being allowed to move. However, he found that Annette really liked it, so he persisted and managed to relax a little more with it the second time.

"Now after practicing it for one week straight I love it!" he said. "It took me a while to overcome my old habits but it's opened up another side to our lovemaking. Annette is prepared to do this more often than normal lovemaking. 'Any time' she says. She really loves it and I guess it's because she enjoys just making love for an hour without having to do anything but enjoy each other."

I asked Annette why she liked the methods, and she said it was because it gives her a lot of time to connect with Allan. They spend a lot of time caressing, holding, kissing, and fondling, so it gives them more time to open up their hearts and feel much more love during lovemaking. There is no performance pressure on either of them and they can enter into it in a relaxed way, being nourished by each other's energy, each other's love.

Annette added: "The other good side of it is I often feel the subtle energy permeating my body throughout the day. Allan says that he feels connected to me all day and that he just can't wait to get back home and make love again."

SOFT ENTRY, HARD WITHDRAWL

If you try these methods a couple of times and you still feel you are getting nothing out of them, then maybe you need to retrain your mind
to appreciate the subtleties in life—the things that give you joy but that
you often take for granted. I also suggest that you do not have sex for
one week. Still fondle, kiss, and hold each other every night without
genital contact, then try again. I promise you, you will have no trouble
feeling the energy. What you will have to watch, though, is your conditioning that will make you want to move to climax. You need to
develop the attitude of being able to take an enormous amount of
pleasure and integrate that through your whole body.

Joseph, one of our students, complained that although he liked the
technique he could not stay erect and his lingam kept falling out. I
explained that as long as the juices were present and he and his
partner were exchanging the magnetic energy, then valley orgasm
could still happen.

However, there is a secret to soft entry. You can still make love without an erection. The main thing for a man is to overcome the psychological belief that he is impotent if he does not have an erection. Men
are conditioned to believe that the lingam has to be hard as steel and
go all night. If it isn't they can become very embarrassed. Most men will
not even attempt to make love once they are soft.

However, the soft lingam can be used in wondrous ways to excite
your woman. The secret is to lie in the scissors position (see page 166),
because it is the easiest way to stay in a woman whether you are erect
or soft. Your lover can take the soft penis and stroke around her clitoris,
and often you will start to get an erection once you see her getting
excited. Or when she is moist she can put your soft penis inside her. If
you are in there long enough you may get an erection. If you don't, just
lie in the scissors position. The main thing is to stay relaxed. You can

have a pleasurable experience just being inside; you do not need to have an erection.

If your woman knows her secrets she will tell you that sometimes she likes it when your lingam is soft. My experience is that you may enter soft, but you nearly always come out hard.

Once you know the secret of soft entry there is no barrier to making love at any time. Include soft entry in your range of lovemaking techniques.

7

Practices to Use During Intercourse

The benefits are enormous for any man learning ejaculation control. One major benefit is that longer periods of lovemaking provide more time for intimacy, communication, loving feelings, and greater pleasure, with deeper and stronger orgasms for yourself and increased opportunities for orgasm for your woman. This doesn't mean, however, that all your lovemaking has to take place over extended periods of time.

A QUICKIE CAN BE FUN

In our workshops Diane and I sometimes ask couples to divide into separate male and female groups. One group of men is asked to discuss some of their fantasies. One recurring fantasy theme is that sometimes a man would like to penetrate his woman and climax without any warmup, because it can be exhausting having to bring her to orgasm first every time.

You might like to make a "quickie" part of the lovemaking repertoire that you share with your beloved. If you are both wanting to open more to love and sexuality, you can set up a situation where one night your woman fulfills any requests that you have and you do the same for her. A quickie might be your request. Your beloved, out of her love for you, honors your request, even though she might not gain any pleasure from it at that moment.

The point is not to concentrate only on long lovemaking periods, but to broaden your range. I liken it to a varied diet. You may savor a long, sit-down, well-prepared meal, but a quick snack on the run can be tasty too. Ejaculation control gives you the same kind of choice.

Another benefit of ejaculation control is that you have more time to absorb the woman's shakti, her energetic essence, which is explained in detail in chapter 9.

Shakti can empower you, rejuvenate you, and heal you. Some men are afraid of losing energy through ejaculation, and some feel drained after they come. However, it is my experience that if you stay in your woman for at least one hour you don't lose energy when you ejaculate, because by then you've absorbed the female essence. By being inside your woman for that length of time you can energetically and psychically absorb this regenerative essence and so balance any loss through ejaculation.

You don't need to pump for the whole sixty minutes. You need to know the secrets of how to fully absorb the essence.

Before you use the following practices in intercourse, discuss them with your beloved and ask her to assist you in practicing ejaculation control.

USE OF THE PC MUSCLE DURING INTERCOURSE

As soon as you experience orgasmic energy during intercourse, clench and hold the PC muscle while simultaneously breathing in. It is vital that you do not wait until the last minute, when all the muscles have tensed up and you are about to ejaculate. You might have done this while you were pleasuring yourself because it was easier, but now it's crucial to stop much earlier in your lovemaking, when you feel the first sensations of the energy building up.

Both partners will need to stop all movement in the early stages of training. You should focus your attention on tightening the PC muscle and remain still. Breathe slowly and deeply, and on the out-breath spread the energy from the lingam throughout your body while relaxing any other muscles that have started to contract. After the urgency to ejaculate has passed you can start moving again.

I would reiterate that it's most important to do your contraction very early during your lovemaking, when you first feel the slightest urge to ejaculate. You may need to do only one strong contraction to move the energy out of the genitals.

If the strong PC contraction doesn't seem to be working, then try to imagine as you are drawing up the muscle that you are sipping your partner's nectar through the head of your lingam, like sipping through a straw, taking the energy right up to the top of your spine. Try breathing in with a strong sipping sound as you draw up the muscle, taking a stream of cool air through your lips. On the out-breath, as you release the muscle imagine the energy spreading out of the genitals, down the legs, and through your entire body.

Initially you may need to do the PC muscle contractions and/or the PC muscle and breath-sipping techniques many times throughout your lovemaking, but as you get more proficient at this skill you will find that two or three times in a lovemaking session is usually enough. Until you get to this stage keep practicing, because it will work for you as it has for hundreds of men with whom I have shared these secrets.

PUMPING THE PROSTATE

The prostate is a muscular gland the size and shape of a chestnut. It is located inside the body behind the scrotum, toward the anus. As you become sexually stimulated it engorges with sexual fluids until, at ejaculation, it pumps its secretions out of the body and is relieved.

The aim of this technique is to relieve the swelling before ejaculation. Providing you begin pumping well before a peak is reached and you pump frequently and firmly, your climax can be delayed as long as you wish.

You can pump the prostate by using the PC muscle once it is

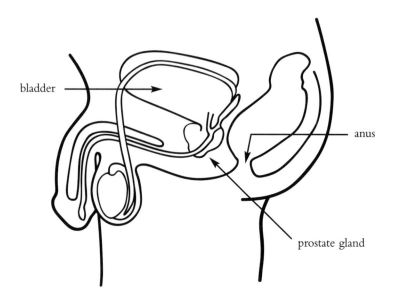

MALE SEXUAL ANATOMY

strong, or you can do it manually. Reach around with three fingers and press deeply and firmly in the area between the anus and the base of the penis and pump it several times. When you apply deep pressure to this area you exert pressure on the prostate, which alleviates the urge to ejaculate.

This point, midway between the anus and the base of the penis, is the perineum. If your touch is sensitive enough you can feel a small indentation in this spot. Pressuring this point relieves the urgency to ejaculate. It has the added benefit of allowing you to keep moving.

I really enjoy it when Diane presses this point for me. One word of warning: if you are not accustomed to your woman touching you in this area, or if you are young, virile, and feeling very horny, or if you have left it to the last minute, pressing on this point may have exactly the opposite effect—that is, it may trigger ejaculation. Pressing early enough is the key to success.

I introduced this secret to a friend of mine and he said it worked, but he had difficulty with it because he lost some of his erection. I reassured Jack that he shouldn't worry about the diminishing of his erection. When the energy moves from the lingam a man will normally lose about 20 percent of his erection, so don't freak out about it. Men panic because they fear not being able to maintain an erection, especially if it has happened to them before. Try to accept that when this happens you are in control and acknowledge yourself for it: "I have the ability to move my energy; I'm getting better at this technique now." This attitude gives you a sense of control over your penis and very soon your erection will return, often stronger than before. It's a big help if your woman knows how to contract her vaginal muscles to help your erection return.

If you reach a point where you are about to ejaculate and you still wish to continue lovemaking and retain the energy, then you'll need to have a well-practiced PC muscle. It's very easy once the PC muscle strengthens. By simply drawing back on the muscle your ejaculation will be reversed. However, if the PC muscle is not strong at this stage you'll have to practice a more powerful technique, such as the breathing sequence where you sip, use the PC muscle, and breathe at the same time (see chapter 5). This is usually powerful enough to take away the urge to ejaculate.

Remember to tell your lover what you are intending to do or she might think you are having a fit or are on some sort of drug. One guy told me he'd read a yoga book that told him to roll his eyes back in his head, press his tongue deep to the roof of his mouth, and clench his teeth to avoid ejaculating. Can you imagine what that must have looked like to his woman?!

Another man told me he practiced a similar technique of drawing the energy up. His woman liked it for the first few months because she could make love to him much longer, but eventually she got to a point where every time he drew back the energy she felt he was doing his own thing and she was just an object. I wouldn't use this strong drawing up and clenching the upper body technique all the time—it's only for emergencies, and your woman should be attuned to that understanding.

TAKING IT TO THE HEART

One of the greatest secrets I can share with you is the technique of "taking it to the heart," because this opens you more to love.

Like most men, I have no trouble feeling sexually excited while lovemaking.

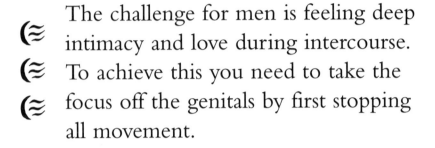

The challenge for men is feeling deep intimacy and love during intercourse. To achieve this you need to take the focus off the genitals by first stopping all movement.

Connect with your partner through your heart and your eyes. Keeping eye contact, look deep into her eyes while you breathe into your chest, at the heart region, and try to feel a deep appreciation of your partner. If it is a person you deeply love, try to bring up as much of that feeling as you can.

Reach out and touch her face or her arm with a sense that every touch is precious. As you are touching, feel the compassion, feel the love for this woman. Say to her: "I love you." Bring the energy from the genitals up into the heart area, where you experience compassion, caring, and nurturing.

You may experience a profound feeling of intimacy because the energy that has been centered around your genitals may move up into the heart area and that feeling can be quite intense. It's like your heart is throbbing with the same sensation that your lingam was. The feeling in your heart can be that of literally burning for your beloved.

You may remember feeling this intense burning sensation after a deep relationship broke up and you really wanted that person back. This is the type of sensation you are trying to achieve to get a sense of deep heart connection and love for the woman you are with. Eye contact

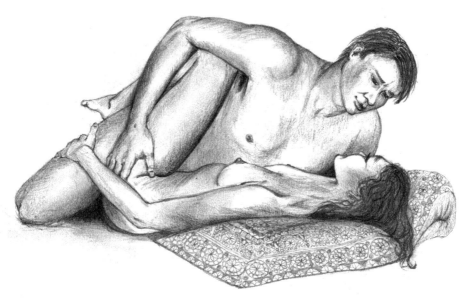

TAKING IT TO THE HEART

helps this because when your eyes are connected you are totally present in your intimacy; you are not off in some other space with your eyes closed.

When your eyes are closed it's delightful to lose yourself in the sensations. However, eyes open creates intimacy, and that's what you are allowing to happen. It might feel uneasy at first but this is the skill, the technique, that turns sexing into lovemaking; your beloved will respond superbly to feeling so deeply loved.

MOVING ENERGY TO YOUR HEART

To assist you in moving the energy to the heart, place your palm at the level of your heart in the center of your chest, the heart chakra. This is traditionally the energy center of the body where you feel love. With your hand on the heart center breathe into this area while focusing your thoughts on your feelings for the woman you are with. This is usually enough to get the energy up into the heart and out of the genitals for this moment.

Another technique for is to place your hands on each other's heart area. Take your beloved's hand and place it on your chest area to feel your own heart. Then take your own hand and place it on her heart area in the center of her chest. Connect eyes again and breathe to the heart region, feeling your compassion, sending your love, and receiving her love.

Tell your woman you love her while receiving and sending your love gently through the eyes, through the heart. Let your hand be an extension of your heart and transmit your love through it.

This practice helps to move the energy that was accumulating in your lingam—and that may have led to ejaculation—to a climax in the heart. The energy isn't as strong in the genitals anymore, and so you can continue to make love longer. The opposite is happening for the woman. Because her heart has been touched the energy in her sexual center becomes more open, balancing the energies for the meeting of the fire and the water.

I introduced this method to a student of ours and his wife. After a month Colin told me that it had been working successfully for him, and that Helen really loved it. He hadn't realized that he and Helen had always made love with their eyes shut. They had been very much into their sexual excitement but had not been emotionally connected to each other.

TRUTH IN THE EYES

During lovemaking it is common to shut our eyes to lose ourselves in the feeling, and that is fine. However, with eyes closed we are often not present with our lover, feeling the intimacy. Shutting the eyes may have something to do with negative programing from the past, where we felt guilty because we were so sexually excited. Most people do not realize how deeply conditioned they have been by society and their parents.

We shut our eyes so we can go off into some space where it is okay to have these sorts of feelings. This may be especially true for women. Young girls are not supposed to show strong sexual feelings.

When we open our eyes during lovemaking it often feels quite awkward at first—to be totally present as a fully opened, sexual, loving, passionate human being and allowing that to be seen by a partner.

Colin told us that making eye contact produced a totally different feeling for Helen and him. They realized that in a lot of their love-making they had not allowed enough intimacy. "Looking into each other's eyes really brought up a sense of truth for us, and at first it was a little threatening. We continued to practice and now we really love it. I especially enjoy seeing the love in Helen's eyes; it's so nur-turing for me and she said she feels much closer to me too. There has been a difficulty, though. Sometimes when Helen is moving on top of me, getting more and more excited, I really don't want to have to stop her, and she doesn't want to stop anyway. So I often don't say anything and we just continue. Sometimes it's okay using the other techniques, but at other times I'll climax before her and then she gets upset. What should I do in these situations?" I told Colin to focus even more on his heart and on his loving feelings for Helen, to repeat to himself while she is moving, "I love you, I love you, Helen," to say it over and over in his own mind—or he can whisper it to her while focusing on his compassion and deep love for her.

"Taking it to the heart" is a fabulous technique. It brings more love into the lives of couples who are in a committed relationship and want to continue to feel love and sexual passion for a lifetime together. Even if you are not in a fully committed relationship this is a great way to bring up feelings of respect and nurturing and care, so that when you are in a committed relationship your heart energy will already be open and you will be ready for love when it comes your way.

You might think that it is natural that when you are with someone you love you feel that love automatically when you are having sex, but this is not necessarily true. Sex is a different arena from love, and couples can get totally lost in sexual feelings. That's all very well, but if you can bring that intensity of feeling into your heart at the same time it generates an even richer experience.

This is what you are doing with this practice. I want to emphasize this most valuable sexual secret for men. This skill has had the most profound effect on my lovemaking. I believe that if I mention it often enough there is a greater chance that you will practice it and use it instead of just reading about it!

THE TESTICLE PULL

Another technique you can use during lovemaking is the testicle pull. "I would rather be punched in the face than have my balls squeezed," you might say, but ball squeezing is not what I'm talking about.

In this technique you hold the scrotum in your hand and pull on the area just above the place where the sac meets the lingam. The testes themselves are held in the hollow of your hand and are not squeezed at all. You pull the whole sac gently and firmly for ten to twenty seconds. You'll be surprised how firmly you can pull without causing any discomfort; this technique actually creates a tension release when you are highly excited.

You would have noticed when you were doing your self-pleasuring exercise that as you became more and more excited and closer to climax your testes started to elevate. During intercourse try this technique of stopping and pulling them down for a while, holding them, and then releasing and starting movement again.

Sometimes when you reach down to delay ejaculation the testes are difficult to find because they have been drawn up inside your body. Pulling down on the testes reverses the process of normal ejaculation. As you get more experienced you can hold them back or have your lover hold them back for you while you continue to move, which is a great advantage of this technique.

A participant in one of our workshops said the technique did not work for him at all. In fact, the act of his woman touching the scrotum excited him more and caused him to ejaculate. I pointed out to Tom that the best thing was to pull down on the testes much earlier. If you are not used to being touched in this area and you leave it until the last moment, then when a woman does touch you it can be the final thing to move you to climax. The idea is to do it much earlier. You could also try it on yourself first a few times before your partner does it for you.

MASTERS AND JOHNSON'S SQUEEZE TECHNIQUE

A more drastic technique that works every time is to completely withdraw from the yoni, then either you or your partner squeeze the frenulum, located about 1 inch from the tip of the lingam. Squeeze firmly on this extremely sensitive area with one finger bent under the head of the penis and the thumb behind the head of the penis. Squeeze and hold until your erection subsides, then reenter and continue.

I used this technique when I was younger, before I had strengthened the PC muscle and before I knew about breath and muscle release. The value of the technique is that it definitely works for anyone without experience in ejaculation control; however, it interrupts the flow of intercourse, and this is a disadvantage.

A MEDITATION TECHNIQUE

This technique was taught to Diane and me by the late Larry Collins. A tantric teacher from San Francisco with a Buddhist background, Larry taught us the power of meditation during lovemaking. The basic idea is that throughout intercourse you are in a deep state of meditation, totally present with everything that is happening—"not missing the valleys" as Larry would put it.

This technique involves three aspects—breath release, thought release, and muscle release. The technique is practiced in a very relaxed and sensitive style. It is a technique Diane and I love very much because it allows for our full emotional and mental presence without any pressure to perform.

MEDITATIVE LOVEMAKING

Begin to make love very slowly. Any extraneous thoughts are gently swept across the mind and not given any attention. Breathe in the essence of the experience with the in-breath and release it through the entire body on the out-breath: "Aahhh!" This continues indefinitely, with no beginning and no end, throughout the your lovemaking; continuously remind yourself of your breath whenever your mind wanders. There is no hurry. You are not going anywhere, you are just trying to remain totally present in the moment—absorbing every sensation, every smell, every feeling, absorbing the energy. This ejaculation-control technique can help you continue to make love for as long as you wish.

NONEJACULATION PRACTICES

Having intercourse but not ejaculating may at first seem like a strange practice. A lot of people ask, "Why make love then? Ejaculating is the best part!" The truth is, ejaculation appears to be the best part of lovemaking only until you learn how to experience other forms of orgasm.

The technique of nonejaculation offers some great benefits. After ejaculation you often feel wasted or tired or you feel a need to eat because a loss of energy has occurred.

Dr. Stephen Chang, a Chinese Taoist master and author of the book *The Tao of Sexology*, says he does not know why orgasm is called "coming." To him it appears to be more like going. The usual rhythm for most lovers is coming, coming, coming, bang, going, going, going. The great disadvantage of this is that the woman is often left frustrated while you have "gone," especially if she has not come.

Even when she has peaked a woman usually remains very open after orgasm because she doesn't lose energy, she gains energy from orgasm. She might release tension and be relaxed, but her energy is high and great to be around. She often enjoys continuing to cuddle, to be intimate, and to talk about love, whereas the man tends to just close down—not only physically but also emotionally—after ejaculation. Sometimes men lose interest altogether, leaving their partners feeling devastated. This sort of behavior can scar a woman for life sexually.

A sexually aware man will continue to hold and cuddle his partner for a while because he understands his woman's needs and not because it is a burning desire for himself. His burning desire for lovemaking happens *before* intercourse; a woman's can often happen *after* intercourse. If you can add nonejaculation to your repertoire of lovemaking skills, you will find your energy level is still very high after a lovemaking session.

Experiment by making love without ejaculating one evening and then go out to dinner together. You will be totally open, sexy, and loving all night, which your woman will love. When you come home you will find you are not tired but full of passion, full of love, full of desire. If you make love again practicing nonejaculation, by the next morning your lovemaking session will be like your very first time. Practice again and you will go off to work charged with energy throughout the entire day. This is of great benefit if you are an older person or your sexual energy is not as strong as your woman's. By the morning she has had three sessions and you are still charged and excited for the next session. There will be no problem getting a strong erection.

The Chinese sex experts who practice the ancient Taoist art of love and sex consider their knowledge and methods of nonejaculation the most important secret men can know for lovemaking. The Taoists believe that the semen *(ching)* is man's most important lifeforce energy. Their belief is that semen is the seed that generates life, so by reversing the process of expelling the seed you can regenerate your own life.

Once a man has ejaculated he feels flat, especially if he ejaculates with great frequency. The Chinese believe that if a man ejaculates too often for his age and health he can experience headaches, lethargy, unclear thinking, and a feeling of distance from his woman; and if he continues squandering his semen he could eventually get very sick.

In 1987, Jolan Chang, in the book *The Tao of Love and Sex,* quoted Taoist master Sun S'sû Mo, the most prominent physician of the Tang period (C.E. 618–906).

> When a man is in his youth
> He usually does not understand the Tao.
> Or even if he does hear or read about it,
> He is not likely to believe it fully and practise it.
> When he reaches his venerable old age,
> He will however realise the significance of the Tao.
> But by then it is often too late,
> For he is usually too sick to benefit fully from it.

In his book Jolan relates that when he was young he tried to follow modern sexuality research, which emphasized simultaneous orgasm. After making love this way three times a day he became very tired; several months later he was sick. It took twelve years before Jolan decided to follow the Taoist advice of nonejaculation. Now he is over sixty, the age when most men make love a lot less frequently, and yet he claims he makes love several times a day.

"Now I am nearly sixty, the age many men have stopped making love entirely. Yet unless I am traveling alone I usually make love several times a day. Often on a Sunday I make love two or three times in the morning and then go cycling for nearly the whole day, about twenty or thirty miles, and then make love again before going to sleep. I am not in the least exhausted, and my health could not be better or my mind more tranquil. And above all, the helpless situation of lying beside an unsatisfied mate no longer exists.

"What is the reason for this change? The answer is that I now practice what the Taoist physician Sun S'sû Mo prescribed 1300 years ago: 'Love one hundred times without emission.'"

This belief that ejaculation robs a man of precious substances necessary for his physical and spiritual well-being is found in many sources of literature, from Taoist works to ayurvedic medical texts and the thirteenth-century Hasidic marriage manual. They all claim that excessive semen loss causes damage to the nervous system, premature aging, muscle weakness, poor digestion, dimmed eyesight, and loss of energy.

In *The Tao of Sexology* Dr. Stephen Chang claims:

> When the average man ejaculates, he loses about one tablespoon of semen. According to scientific research, the nutritional value of this amount of semen is equal to that of two pieces of New York steak, ten eggs, six oranges, and two lemons and a lime. That includes proteins, minerals, vitamins, amino acids, everything. The semen also contains a great deal of vital energy. Therefore an ejaculation also represents a great deal of loss of vital energy. This is demonstrated by the exhaustion felt by the man after ejaculation.

In contemporary research there has been controversy over whether or not excessive semen loss results in ill health. Certainly it is recognized that semen loss often results in a loss of energy—that is why athletes are warned not to have intercourse before an important event. What they should be told is to not ejaculate. Making love actually charges the energy.

My advice to athletes would be to make love before an event, but to retain the energy through nonejaculation and to integrate that energy within the body. Then they will have more energy for sport, not less.

The medical profession claims that semen loss makes little difference to a man's health because the body reproduces the semen again. This is true, but it takes lifeforce to produce that semen again.

My feeling is that the more you use up this lifeforce, the faster you age. If you are continually fighting an illness, for example, it eventually drains you. I feel that this is the same for an older man who continually forces himself to ejaculate. It draws on his reserves and ages him quickly. Obviously there is disagreement on the value of nonejaculation. All I can do is refer to my personal experience and to the people who practice nonejaculation. They speak highly of the benefits and are unusually vital and very active for their age. Napoleon Hill, in his classic bestseller *Think and Grow Rich,* refers to seminal conservation, praising it as one of the greatest success secrets a man has at his command.

It was the Taoist writings that convinced me that it was worth trying. I decided that Taoist culture, which for thousands of years treated sexuality as one of the highest forms of study, had more long-term experiences to draw on than the more recent Western research into sexology, which only looks at how the body reproduces semen and therefore assumes nonejaculation has no benefit.

Another benefit of nonejaculation is that it helps to remedy the times when your sex drive is not as strong as your partner's. This is a great problem for some men, but there is a very simple solution. All you need to do is practice nonejaculation several times and you will find your energy coming back. It means you can make love, but you do not ejaculate every time. Psychologically it means changing your mind-set about this.

If you think the only way you can have intercourse is when it culminates in ejaculation then it is a matter of educating your mind, and your woman's, about the process. Very often women believe that if you do not ejaculate then they have not fully satisfied you. Believe me, your partner will soon forgive you once she starts to see the benefits of nonejaculation. When you discover that orgasm is not dependent upon ejaculation, you will benefit from the tremendous experiences it will open up to you.

Another benefit of ejaculation control is that, when you make love the second and third time after nonejaculation, you will be amazed at how good it feels when you do come. You will feel eighteen again and the climax will be very powerful.

Another benefit is for older people, who, as they are having less sex, are not getting the amount of loving and touching they need. When you can make love more, without the pressure to perform every time, you can build up your energy and you'll find that you feel more love for each other. Love is a healing force. You can rejuvenate your body, not only by not using up your vital energy but also by receiving more touching and more loving.

TOO MUCH FOCUS ON NONEJACULATION

You can go over the top with some of these practices. My own experience is that too much concentration on the nonejaculation technique creates tightness. Some books suggest ejaculating only once every hundred times you make love. I once practiced nonejaculation for a period of three years. I would ejaculate only once every five or ten times. I found I became very uptight and I noticed other people who had practiced that way becoming tense too. When they did come they felt guilty and did not enjoy it. Mentally they were telling themselves that by ejaculating they were aging. After orgasm the mind is very receptive, and these thoughts can program the mind. If you keep telling yourself you're aging you will cause the body to age.

I advise you to acknowledge the benefits of nonejaculation but don't become fanatical about it. At first, practice it once in every five or so lovemaking sessions. To determine how often to practice, listen closely to your body and your responses. If you feel tired and drained after you have ejaculated, then the next time you make love you should not ejaculate. If you feel charged and energized, then the next time you make love there is nothing wrong with ejaculating. Allow your own physical lifeforce to determine how often you use this technique. Even if you rarely have a problem with energy it is still a good idea to start practicing nonejaculation now, so that when you are older you will be proficient.

For those who practice nonejaculation regularly and are experiencing the benefits but also some of the difficulties, I recommend you to try another practice and see how it makes you feel. Accepting that there is a physical loss and an energy loss when you ejaculate, it is my experience that this loss can be balanced by "drawing off" the essence of the semen. At the point of climax, instead of ejaculating try to draw off, or reabsorb, the essence using the breath and the PC muscle-contraction technique. Spread that essence throughout your body. You are actually taking lifeforce into your body. Absorbing the essence is like drawing up the steam of the substance. I call it "steaming off the essence of the semen." What is left is like waste product. If you experience the reabsorption of this essence several times and then ejaculate, you will often find your energy has been balanced. What has been lost physically has been regained energetically through the absorption of the essence.

PELVIC CONGESTION RELIEF

If you choose to practice nonejaculation, at some stage you will need to be familiar with congestion relief. After making love using the nonejaculation technique you may experience pain in the scrotum or a swelling in that area.

You need to lie down and pump your perineum by pressing firmly with your fingers on the area midway between your anus and the base of your penis. This massages the prostate gland. Press firmly on this area at least one hundred times. Your partner can do this for you too. Alternately you can use the breath and PC muscle-squeeze technique. Hold the PC muscle firmly as you hold your breath. As you release the breath and the PC muscle imagine the energy spreading out of the prostate and throughout your whole body, especially along the arms and legs.

Another method involves pulling the scrotum down while having a shower so that the warm water runs around that area. Hold the scrotum down and continually rub your lower abdomen below the navel in a circular motion at the same time. Every morning in the shower I practice pulling the scrotum down equal to the number of years of my age. This is also an ancient technique for strength of erection and longevity. You could make this a regular practice in the shower.

Another method is to sleep with a hot water bottle around this area.

You might think that all this is just not worth it! But remember that the benefits of being able to make love more often, being able to satisfy your woman more, of having more powerful experiences yourself and not feeling drained and tired after intercourse all far outweigh the chore of pelvic-congestion relief.

A few words of advice. If you find nonejaculation difficult you might need to make some dietary changes. Perhaps you are eating a lot of foods that contain chemicals and additives, or perhaps you have a high meat intake and your blood is hot. Experiment with changing your diet for one month and see what happens; for example, cut down on your meat intake, eat more fresh fruit and vegetables, and eat less processed food.

If you have any form of prostate trouble you should not practice this technique until your condition clears. As well, nonejaculation can aggravate nonspecific urinary-tract infections. You need to clear up these conditions first before practicing the techniques described in this book. Some excellent remedies for these problems can be found in Chinese medicine or homeopathy, and these remedies have few side effects.

8

Satisfying a Woman on Every Level

One of our students told me that he had mastered the techniques of ejaculation control and was confident of being able to make love for as long as he wished. He was really pleased with himself because now his partner had an orgasm nearly every time they made love. Interestingly, his girlfriend had told Diane that she was not feeling totally satisfied with their lovemaking. Tina said: "I love the sex and it's wonderful now that Tim goes long enough for me to build up to orgasm. However, I feel there is still something missing. It's hard to describe, but I just don't feel fully nourished. I feel good and I feel satisfied sexually, but I don't feel we are any closer—and the next day it seems like our lovemaking never happened. I hoped our lovemaking would connect us more in our day-to-day life, but it doesn't seem to bring us any closer."

Women often express this difficulty to Diane. Although they are being satisfied on one level, on another level something seems to be missing. What can you do about this? The solution is to learn what I call the art of energic lovemaking. This is where you not only enjoy the physical connection between you and your partner, but there is also a focus on the exchange of love and sexual energy passing between you both. It is a method of lovemaking that has healed many relationships, especially in marriages where sex had become only a small part of something the partners shared together, as opposed to the most beautiful way to bond with one another.

Energic lovemaking is probably a softer style of sex than you are accustomed to. Ordinary sex is what I call "hard sex." It tends to engage in love from a physical perspective, placing the focus on sexual pleasure and orgasm. It emphasizes physical characteristics—a good body, good looks, strong movement, and jubilant response. It is usually intense and fast-moving, with lots of banging and pumping. This is the form of sex we see in movies and read about in novels. Hard sex can be fulfilling and fun and should be part of your lovemaking repertoire, but if it is the only method you rely on to give you pleasure then your woman may end up dissatisfied and perhaps eventually you will, too.

If anyone else ever gives her an experience like I'm going to share with you, you can be sure she will want more of the same. If you are not the one who nourishes her, she will soon find someone who will.

If you can include in the range of ways you make love with your woman at least one energic lovemaking session per week she'll never want to leave you, because very few men know anything of this form of lovemaking. Most men know about the clitoris and the G-spot and all the positions, about how to pump well, and about softness and gentleness in foreplay, but once they enter the yoni their old programs start to take over. They pump faster and their mind goes faster: "I must not come too soon," "I must give her a good time so she'll know I'm a good lover," "I must bring her to orgasm." The tension starts to build, the movements start to build, the breath starts to build, there's a lot of fast pumping—their eyes are shut and they are doing a good job. This is normal sex for most people—it's physical and hard.

However, you can make a choice not to be "normal" in bed. You can choose to be extraordinary in bed. How? Let's take a look at lovemaking from an energy perspective rather than just a physical perspective. Start to focus on the energy exchange during lovemaking.

I'm not suggesting this is the only way to make love. I'm saying that if you add it to the range of ways you express your love, you will be a better lover than the average man.

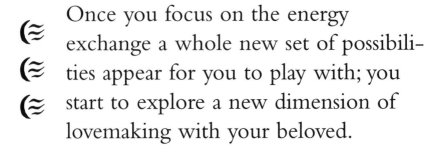 Once you focus on the energy exchange a whole new set of possibilities appear for you to play with; you start to explore a new dimension of lovemaking with your beloved.

LOVEMAKING FROM AN ENERGY PERSPECTIVE

Modern physics maintains that all things consist of energy vibrating at different frequencies. When you make love your energy fields merge and weave together. These energy fields or auras have been photographed through Kirlian photography. In a Kirlian photograph, when two people send out negative thoughts to each other the energy bodies separate. When they send loving thoughts the energy bodies merge; it is hard to tell where one energy body finishes and the other starts. That is why sometimes when you are making love you and your lover can feel like one body. A feeling of harmony arises when your energy body resonates at the same frequency as your beloved's. Some say our etheric bodies merge.

Energic lovemaking will be quite new to most people, just as this energetic view of the world is relatively new in science. The process of understanding ourselves as energy beings is in its infancy. However, Hindu, Chinese, and Aboriginal traditions for centuries have focused on understanding humans as energy beings. The Hindu system refers to the lifeforce as *kundalini* or *shakti*. The Chinese call it *chi*. It's also called sexual energy, psychic energy, physical energy, nervous energy, spiritual energy, light, and lifeforce. How we use and experience energy determines what we call it.

The Hindus and the Chinese believe that this lifeforce is stored like a reservoir at the base of the spine and is our infinite source of spiritual energy. It is represented as a sleeping serpent, a representation that has spiritual and sexual meanings. When you dream of snakes you are tapping in to your spiritual and sexual energies and awakening them. In the Hindu system the aim is to awaken the kundalini energy in the sexual center and move it to the higher centers of the body, to expand your consciousness and lead you into enlightenment, or a tangible experience of God. You can awaken it by yourself and move it through these centers to create a high state of meditation. Awakening the kundalini as an individual and raising it up through the sexual center to all the other centres is called white tantra.

When a couple comes together to awaken the sexual and spiritual energy by meditating together in union in order to reach a heightened state of awareness it is called red tantra. This is one of the quickest ways to awaken the kundalini energy. I find red tantra a much more powerful meditative experience than white tantra, which I practiced for many years. Men and women are perfectly created as complementary polar opposites. When a man and a woman come together a circuit is set up, and unlimited energy is available to you.

The ancient Chinese said that man's energy is like fire while woman's energy is like water. If you do not practice the sexual secrets, water will put out fire every time. In other words, as you ejaculate your fire goes out but the water continues to flow. Those practiced in the art of lovemaking know that coming together is not about putting out the fire but rather warming the woman's water until it steams. That steam rises and fills you both with energy through your entire bodies. When you make love in this way you focus not only on the physical sensations but also on the energy exchange between you. This gives you a totally different experience in your lovemaking.

When working with energy it is important to understand the main energy centers of your body. Just as your physical organs determine your physical well-being, so your energy centers determine your energetic well-being. As explained earlier, there are seven chakras that occur vertically along the spine. The first chakra is located at the base of the spine and is considered to be the center that deals with basic survival instincts. The seventh chakra, located at the crown, is believed to be the link to the spiritual plane. Between these two are the second chakra, in the nerve plexus above the genitals, relating to instincts and sexual passion; the third chakra, in the solar plexus, relating to emotions and willpower; the fourth chakra, the heart, relating to love and compassion; the fifth chakra, in the thyroid gland, relating to self-expression, communication, and creativity; and the sixth chakra, in the middle of the forehead between the eyebrows, relating to intuition, insight, and vision.

Throughout your daily life certain energy centers close down or resonate at a lower frequency than your partner's, while other energy centers open and become overactive. When you come together to make love you are often not on the same frequency. Perhaps through the day you may have dealt with some negative people or been exposed to bad news in the media. You close down in the heart area a little in order to protect yourself. Meanwhile your partner may have dealt with a different set of problems that required a lot of thinking and decision making. Because of this her energies will be very much in the head, vibrating at a high frequency, with very little energy in the emotional and physical centers.

When you come together to make love you will be completely out of harmony. You will be lucky if even at the end of your lovemaking session your energy centers have started to harmonize. But if you have a high sexual experience then at least the sexual centers will be harmonized.

However, when you look at lovemaking from an energetic perspective, part of the focus of your lovemaking is to harmonize all your energy centers during lovemaking, or, even better, before you actually get into bed together. There are ways to do this, as I'll explain below. I will also give you a step-by-step guide to the art of energic lovemaking. Try it the next time you make love and you'll find you can nourish and satisfy your woman on every level of her being.

Sexual energy combined with visualization is a great way to increase the rate of vibration in any of the chakras. One aspect of energic lovemaking involves harmonizing these energy centers so that they resonate with your partner's. To harmonize the vibrations you send energy to each other psychically, using visual focus and breath aware-ness. You can amplify the energy by pumping the PC muscle, which releases the kundalini.

ENERGIC LOVEMAKING TECHNIQUES

The following technique will help you to harmonize energies with your partner so you feel nourished on every level. It's an especially good tech-nique for harmonizing the sexual centers when there is an imbalance in libido between partners. It works well for sexual difficulties such as impo-tence, premature ejaculation, frigidity, and reduced sexual drive. In any of these cases this technique should be practiced every day for a week, and then at least twice a week after that. Even if you are older and have not had sex for a while, this practice will awaken and restore your sexual drive.

One of our students introduced this technique to his seventy-year-old father, who had just remarried and had trouble keeping up with his seventy-five-year-old wife. The imbalance in their sexual energies was causing him stress. His father commented: "It's a great position because I don't have to have the old feller hard to stay inside."

This is the best technique to use to stay inside your woman, even when you are not erect. The warmth and moisture are sure to turn you on after a while. His father said, "If it's not the first day, then by the third day of using this technique I'm hard and ready to get on top again. Sometimes while I'm soft inside her she stimulates herself to orgasm and that always makes the old feller stand up again."

THE SCISSORS

The woman lies on her back and you lie at an angle to her on your right side. Both should be comfortable. You may wish to put a pillow under your head. The woman puts her right leg between your legs and her left leg over your hip in a scissors position. Your lingam, whether hard or soft, is inserted into her yoni. If it is quite flaccid then press it against the vaginal opening.

No physical movement is made throughout the practice. To begin, both of you are relaxing, attuning, feeling. Both focus on the genital area. Close your eyes and visualize an orange sphere of energy in your sexual center radiating energy like the sun. Send that energy through your lingam into your partner's body. This starts to awaken the kundalini, the sexual and spiritual energy.

Inhale, drawing up and squeezing the PC muscle. As you exhale send the energy through your lingam into your partner's body, through her yoni to the crown of her head. Then inhale again, pulling the energy back from your partner's crown through her sexual organs all the way up to your crown. Your partner is doing the same, psychically mixing her energy with yours.

After picturing the energy flowing back and forth for several minutes, relax and tune in to the feelings in your bodies while entering a meditative state. Continue meditating together in this way for about thirty minutes. This technique aligns the seven chakras of the male with

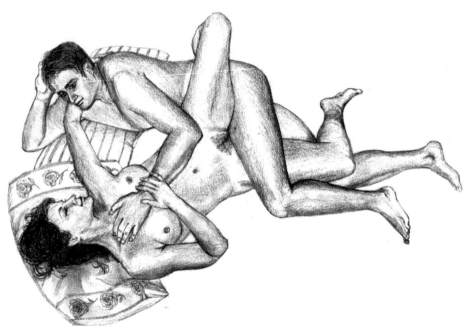

THE SCISSORS

the seven chakras of the female and heightens the awareness of each to the combined energies.

If you want to make love in your usual way before or after using this technique by all means do so, but during the technique there is no movement except for a contraction of the vaginal muscles every now and then to maintain the erection. The focus is on the energy exchange rather than the physical striving for orgasm.

Some students have described their energic lovemaking experience as a sense of transcending their bodies, a feeling of two energies merging and becoming one, a bonding emotionally, physically, and mentally, the same sense that can be created through deep meditation. Some even describe it as having a sense of oneness or total union with all things.

This next practice helps you to tune in to your partner's energy through your hands. It can be done either sitting on the floor or in chairs opposite one another.

FEELING THROUGH THE HANDS

Both partners sit comfortably face to face, holding hands. Close your eyes, breathe deeply, and relax. Imagine that the only way you have of communicating is through sensing the energy in the hands. Each person relaxes and tries to pick up the feelings of the other.

Next, with eyes closed move your palms about 1.5 inches apart from your partner's palms and sense the energy fields between them. You may feel a warmth or a tingling as you pick up on the energy body. As you become aware you can feel this energy field very strongly between your hands. After three to five minutes of doing this tell each other what you have experienced.

This is the simplest form of energic lovemaking and can be done with anyone, not just your lover, as a way of connecting with them on a deeper level. With your lover it can be used as a preparation for lovemaking.

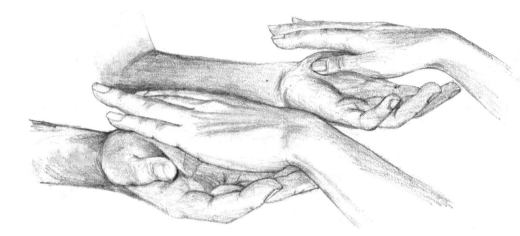

FEELING THROUGH THE HANDS

CHAKRA BREATHING

Both partners sit opposite each other. Close your eyes while your partner sensitively touches each of your chakra centers. As she touches a chakra imagine that center awakening for you. She can amplify the energy by using her PC muscle. As she squeezes she inhales, imagining energy accumulating in her sexual center. As she releases the breath she imagines that energy moving along her arm and out her fingertips and into your energy center. She can amplify the energy by pumping her PC muscle. She repeats this pumping as she touches each chakra.

At the throat center she says: "This is to open your communication to express your true feelings and your true heart's wish."

At the heart center she says: "This is to open your heart to allow in my love."

At the solar plexus area she says: "This is to give you courage, strength, and power in your daily life."

At your sexual center she says: "This is to awaken your sexual pleasure and passion."

Then your partner closes her eyes. You repeat the process for her, remembering to use the PC muscle each time to amplify the energy.

When you have both finished, sit still and gently open your eyes. Coordinate your breathing, maintain eye contact, and focus on the breath to keep your mind present. Say to your partner, "Follow my breathing," and try to breathe together as one body. Keeping eye contact, imagine you are breathing through the third eye. As you breathe in, imagine a vapor coming out from your partner's third eye into your third eye. As you exhale, mix her vapor with yours and send them across through her third eye. Do this for ten to fifteen breaths.

The PC muscle can be used to amplify the energy if you wish. Your partner does the same thing as she inhales and exhales through her third eye. Doing this harmonizes your visions.

Then you do the same from the throat center, the communication center, to harmonize your communication as a couple, from the heart center to harmonize your love, from the solar plexus center to harmonize and mix your power as a couple, and from the sexual center to harmonize your sexual energies so that they resonate at the same frequency.

With this practice you are interpenetrating each other's energy body, mixing your essences so the two of you are becoming one energy body, resonating at the same frequency in each of your energy centers.

Once you have completed the chakra breathing you can move into the next step, which is to harmonize the sexual center with the heart center.

CIRCULATING LOVE AND SEXUAL PASSION

Have your woman place her right hand on your heart center and cup your genitals with her left hand. Place your right hand on her heart center and your left hand on her yoni. This is to awaken your sexual energy and your love at the same time, so that in lovemaking when you are feeling sexual passion you can take that

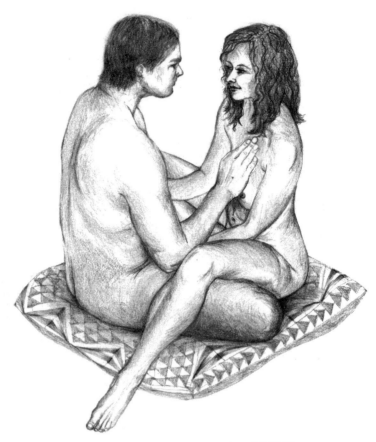

HARMONIZING THE SEXUAL CENTER
WITH THE HEART CENTER

passion to your heart. Not only does she feel the intensity of your sexual passion, but she also receives your feelings of love at the same time. This then becomes special lovemaking, not just sex. Do this for a period of two or three minutes.

If these energy centers have been opened, you can both take your hands away and experience psychic lovemaking, lovemaking without genital contact. You begin by sending energy from your lingam across to your beloved's yoni. As you breathe in, you draw back the energy, mixed with her vaginal essence, into your lingam. Then direct the energy back to her again. To amplify the energy, as you breathe in suck up your PC muscle and as you release your breath let it go. She should feel and sense the energy entering her being.

After a few minutes, sit still and say, "I'm ready to receive." As she sends you her yoni energy on her exhalation see if you can sense the power of her essence entering your lingam, mixing with your essence. Once you have both received, start breathing together so that you are both breathing from lingam to yoni, yoni to lingam, keeping the breaths coordinated, the two becoming one.

Next, extend the exhaled breath and visualize the energy passing from your lingam not only into her yoni but right up to her heart. On your inhalation pull the energy back from her heart, down through her yoni, up through your lingam, and into your heart. Continue mixing your essences like this for a few minutes.

For the next stage your woman sits on your lap facing you. You can sit on a chair, or in a cross-legged position on the floor or bed. The woman may like to place a pillow under her buttocks to take some of the weight off your legs. Keeping your spines straight, insert your lingam into the yoni or touch that area with your lingam. Holding one another, press your heart and sexual centers together, melting into one body. Using the breathing, visualization, and PC-muscle techniques, send the energy from your lingam. Continue to send energy back and forth, but this time send it right up the back of her spine to her tongue, the other nectar center of bodily fluids, while she does the same.

After several cycles inhale together, hold your breath, and touch tongues as you breathe out. You will often feel a spark pass from one tongue to the other. This can be a magic moment if the energy has built up strongly enough. On exhalation release the energy down through each other's body. Your lovemaking becomes a circuit of energy and essence exchange, an inner circle and an outer circle.

Do this for at least ten cycles, then stop and hold each other. Be sensitive to the energy you are creating through your entire body and melt into that energy. Be in the present with hardly any movement—perhaps a little rocking back and forth but be sure to stay in the moment.

Continue this energetic lovemaking session for about forty minutes, varying between breathing cycles and stillness. Remember: the goal is not to orgasm but to be in the moment, to absorb and mix your energy with your beloved's, to experience the valley. The entire session can be orgasmic in a subtle sense.

These four techniques of energetic lovemaking are fine methods of attunement for making love in different ways than you normally do. Obviously it would be delightful to go in to your normal lovemaking after forty minutes. However, to fully appreciate energetic lovemaking give yourself the gift of doing this sequence on its own without turning it into anything else. Afterward, go out to dinner or to a movie and see how you feel being in this energy space. You will feel connected all night. Come back and make love later if you wish.

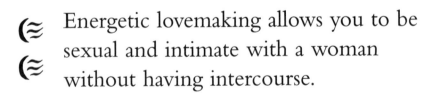 Energetic lovemaking allows you to be sexual and intimate with a woman without having intercourse.

You can even try energetic lovemaking with your clothes on before having sex, especially if you are with a new partner. If this leaves you feeling tense in the genitals, you need to spread the energy through your body using the techniques described earlier. Once you have become familiar with these energetic lovemaking techniques, I suggest you try the following.

A THREE-STEP PRACTICE

Study the following sequence so that the next time you make love you can integrate some of it and see what kind of experience you can create for yourself and your beloved. It may feel a little unusual the first time, but I assure you that after enough practice it will be one of the most wonderful lovemaking sessions you ever experience.

This Energetic Lovemaking sequence is very powerful. It can change your relationship. It can change your entire love life.

Phase 1: Attuning Energies

First, clear out any negative energy you may have brought in from the day—take a shower or a walk to accomplish this. Then come together, sitting back to back. Breathe together by following each other's breath. Use the PC muscle to draw energy up your spine; imagine energy moving up your spine as you inhale and hold. On

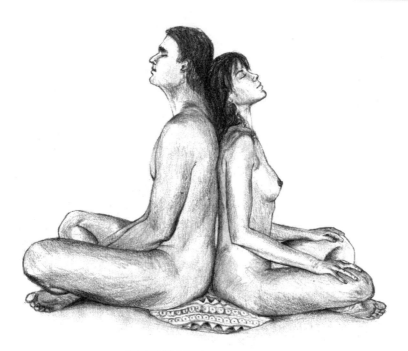

ATTUNING YOUR ENERGY

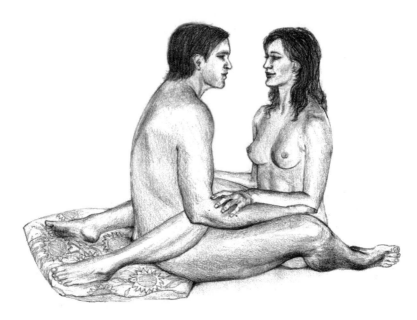

OPENING YOUR HEARTS WITH CHAKRA BREATHING

exhalation release the energy down through the spine. This will coordinate and harmonize your energies. You could look at this as a shared meditation.

Phase 2: Opening the Heart

After a couple of minutes, turn to face each other and gently focus on each other's eyes, the windows to the soul. Coordinate your breathing again. Now is the time to forgive, to heal, to open up. Place your hand on your partner's heart center and say, "May this open your heart to allow my love in." She then does the same to you. The second time you try this include some chakra breathing with this step.

Phase 3: Psychic Lovemaking

With your woman's permission, send your energy and love to her through your lingam. Send energy from your lingam into her yoni using the PC muscle, breath, and visualization and ask her if she is able to feel the energy and the healing and the love you are sending. Then ask her to send her yoni energy to you using her PC muscle. As she does, breathe out and imagine absorbing the energy. Show her how it is affecting you—"Aahhh!"— because this empowers her.

As the energy moves upward in you body, start sending it from your heart to her heart, via the sexual center, in a U shape. Ask her to sit on your lap. Do not rush to have your lingam enter her yoni. Concentrate on cycling the energy through the touching of your tongues. By gently rocking back and forth your lingam may become erect. As it enters the yoni continue the cyclic breathing. Do this for five to ten cycles and then hold and absorb, drinking deeply of the connection. Start caressing, arousing, teasing, playing, and loving.

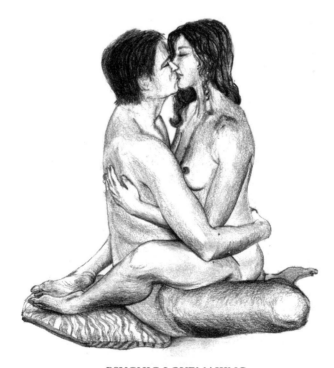

PSYCHIC LOVEMAKING

As your partner's energy builds, allow her to dance on your lingam by moving her hips. You have the ejaculation control methods to allow her to do whatever movement feels good for her. Move with her, then stop at a peak and absorb the energy and enjoy the silence. Build the energy close to climax again and hold that peak. Move once more to a final peak and, as the energy builds, draw it up; drink deeply. Pull your chin in and hold the energy, hold the breath, hold the PC muscle, and ask her to do the same.

Now release and let go. Feel the energy spread throughout your entire body, as if you were being showered in light. If this is as far as you choose to go, then lie down head to feet beside each other and rest your inside hand on each other's heart center and melt into this energy.

Alternatively you may want to complete the session by moving into the position in which your partner normally orgasms or into a position in which you feel comfortable making love. Use your ejaculation-control techniques until she is fully satisfied. Do not be surprised if your partner orgasms many times. Then release either just after or with her, or let her peak you again a couple of more times until finally you release on a deep exhalation. As long as you extend the breath the sensations of the pumping of the PC muscle continue. Lie in the afterglow for at least ten minutes, softly kissing, caressing, holding, and talking.

If you do not complete this sequence exactly or you want to change it around that is fine, but at some time do try to accomplish it. If you do not complete it the first time or it doesn't work, try it again.

This energic lovemaking sequence is very powerful. It can change your relationship. It will change your love life!

For couples who are always exploring new and exciting ways to make love, energic lovemaking broadens the many ways they already

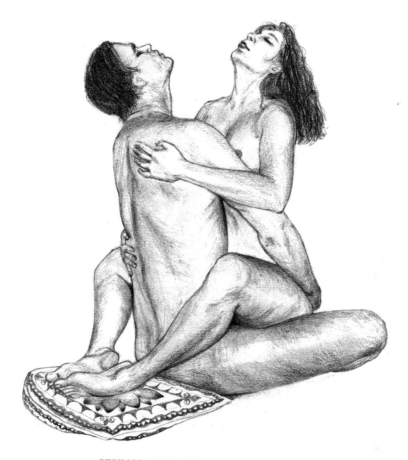

SEXUAL AND SPIRITUAL ECSTASY

connect. For single men who are not in a committed relationship and want to be seen as good lovers, this is one of the most precious things I can share with you. In our workshops I have shared this method with numerous single men who have tried it with their girlfriends and have reported that it totally blows the women away. Many men have reported to me that their partners shed tears of joy. This is because the women have been waiting so long to be loved like this that when it finally happens they release a lot of tension. Energic lovemaking is a terrific technique for nourishing your woman and yourself on every level and for making your lovemaking experience memorable, enjoyable, and special.

IF YOU DON'T HAVE A PARTNER

Practicing these skill-building exercises without a partner presents a difficulty. What you can do without a partner is visualize yourself *with* a partner, using your breath and PC-muscle contractions to send and receive love and sexual energy. This opens up the pathways for the energy to move in your mind and body so that when you *do* have a partner it will flow more easily.

Reading about the lovemaking practices and visualizing yourself using them is an important step. However it is only when you put these into practice with a woman that you get to experience the success of your practice and just how much women like being touched on this deeper spiritual and heartfelt level.

At my men's seminars single men would often express a concern that they didn't have anyone to practice with and were not confident about trying some of these practices with a new lover. Through Diane's women's workshops she had connections with some single women who were skilled in the arts of tantra and were willing to guide in the practices of sacred love. This was only for men who were authentically wanting to learn and willing to meet these women first to see if there was a mutual attraction.

In ancient times there were women who lived in the temples of Aphrodite, the goddess of love and sensuality. They were the temple priestesses who would use their lovemaking skills for healing and transformation, to give a man a tangible experience of the love of the goddess Aphrodite and a connection to the sacred.

A client who had studied with me related this story after a couple of sessions with Jasmine.

"I felt completely nurtured and pampered in the arms of a goddess.
I experienced that I could handle higher levels of pleasure without
fear of ejaculating too soon. I trusted her enough to open my heart
more and she helped me verbalize my feelings. It was invaluable

practice in ways of giving a woman greater pleasure, both physically and emotionally.

"It was a relief to be able to ask questions and get guidance without being put down like had happened to me previously. My marriage of eight years was very difficult for the last three years. My wife was always criticizing me for not lasting long enough and sex was hardly happening between us. After our breakup whenever I met a new woman I would find myself avoiding getting too intimate with her in case she discovered that I wasn't a good lover. Recently I met a lady I really liked and even though I had read about tantra I found myself reticent to introduce her to it. I guess I was afraid of messing it up. However, now that I have had the practice with Jasmine I feel so much more confident about doing tantra with her. It has been an extremely valuable experience for me."

If you so desire you can work with a modern-day goddess of love to put your reading into practice (see "For More Information" page 248). When you do meet a woman with whom you would like to form a long-term relationship you will have developed a quiet sexual confidence about you that will not only be attractive to her but will also allow you both to go on an adventure together into levels of love and sexual pleasure neither of you have explored so far. Something as special as sacred sex can keep the magic of a relationship alive for many years.

9

Shakti Power—The Female Force

Many ancient cultures had traditions that exalted the female force. Woman was considered the embodiment of sensuality and the guardian of the creative force. From her all life came and so the cultures honored her initiatory power. As every human being is born through the yoni, the yoni was worshiped.

Men would go to pray to the yoni in temples where there were huge rocks carved into the shape of a yoni. Today most men appreciate yoni, but praying to it, that's another issue! The yoni was seen as a source of all life. I imagine that women in these ancient cultures felt very good about their yonis and their sexual energy.

In Hindu mythology the goddess Shakti represents the female principle, the female energy. This female force, or shakti, exists in both men and women, but women are the guardians of the shakti energy. In tantric writings a woman's sexual and spiritual energy is often referred to as shakti energy. In tantric writings from ancient India the power of the shakti has no bounds—it is limitless. This spiritual/sexual force, once awakened, brings out the goddess nature in women and empowers them. Once a man and a woman appreciate what the shakti energy is, then as a couple they can source this limitless force, learning to recognize it, awaken it, and channel it creatively.

Woman's shakti energy has been suppressed for more than two thousand years and it is only now reawakening. The first real awakening of the shakti began about thirty years ago when, with the liberation movement, women's energy started to be felt strongly in the world. Women expanded their influence into business, politics, and spiritual pursuits, but this was only the first level of the awakening. Now many women are moving on from the liberation movement toward the awakening of the archetypal goddess or priestess within. This doesn't negate their efforts in business, politics, or other public arenas. They simply use less male energy in these pursuits and focus instead on the interconnectedness and relationship of things, with greater emphasis on ecology than economy.

Soon the true shakti will emerge from within women and heal the world of what is happening to it now. It's a force that must be awakened at this point in our history. Men and women will start to work more with the shakti energy, the feminine energy, in order to create more harmony in the world.

Why was woman's shakti energy suppressed for more than two millennium? One explanation is that man became frightened of the intensity of woman's sexual energy and so suppressed her power. Men and women both need to learn how to rekindle woman's dormant sexual energy and not to be afraid of it, but rather to embrace it and rejoice in it. When a woman awakens her sexual energy, often her spiritual energy is awakened as well. She becomes more in touch with her divine essence, her goddess nature. Some men practice celibacy to reach their spiritual enlightenment, but according to Tantric texts the path to woman's spiritual enlightenment is through the electric charge of her orgasmic energy.

Women are becoming more orgasmic nowadays, more comfortable with their sexual energy, and this is only the beginning of their awakening. Women's orgasmic energy is potentially unlimited.

FEMALE EJACULATION

In sessions we have taught on releasing the orgasm, many women have reported releasing large quantities of a light liquid during orgasm. Yes, women ejaculate! I'm not just talking about the secretions of sexual intercourse. I'm talking about ejaculation.

In ancient writings this substance is called *amrita,* or divine nectar. Where it may have surprised you before to learn that men can orgasm without ejaculation, now I'm saying that women can orgasm with ejaculation. There is some controversy over this, but to those of us who have experienced it there is no doubt because we know what it is and what it looks like.

Most doctors and many sexologists don't acknowledge the existence of female ejaculation, or they say it's simply normal vaginal secretions that occur due to sexual excitement and that some women secrete more than others.

Both Taoist writings from China and tantric writings from ancient India talk about ejaculation in women, as does Galen, a famous second-century physician. In 1672 the Dutch anatomist de Graaf talked about female ejaculation "rushing out," and Van de Velde, in his well-known book, *Ideal Marriage,* points out that women expel a liquid during orgasm, adding that half the men in the world believe this.

A breakthrough in research into human sexuality was made in 1980 by two sex researchers, Dr. John Perry and Beverly Whipple. They documented on film women expelling a clear fluid at the moment of orgasm. Many doctors claimed it was urine and suggested it was simply "urinary incontinence." However, Perry and Whipple did a laboratory analysis and found the secretion was neither urine nor vaginal secretions as other sexologists suggested. It was found to be high in prostatic acid, phosphatase, and gluconal—like male ejaculation—and low in urea and creatinine, unlike urine.

Perry and Whipple found that extended stimulation of the G-spot very often resulted in the release of this fluid. In ancient writings the G-spot was called the "sacred spot" and the liquid was considered a divine nectar. Most women prefer this terminology to the medical terms.

One woman told Diane that when she was young and pleasured herself she nearly always released a fluid at orgasm. But the first time it happened with a man he made some comment like, "You've wet the bed." It embarrassed her so much that she learned to hold it back.

I think this must happen to a lot of women. The sad thing is that such experiences can have the effect of not allowing the woman to really let go during orgasm. Once you let your lover know she has blessed you with divine nectar from her sacred place she will start to feel comfortable about letting go. Sometimes she will let go with laughter, tears, or love. This is a great experience for both of you.

Many women will be glad there is finally a scientific explanation for what they have been experiencing all these years. Where it comes from we are not sure. Biologically the fluid appears to originate in one of the Bartholin glands, which lie on either side of the lower part of the vagina. The ejaculate itself varies in color from clear to slightly opaque. It can taste astringent or sweet or have no taste at all. As it is expelled from the urethra the first drops may have the slightly salty taste of urine.

In my opinion the reason a lot of women don't experience the release of the fluid, the amrita, is that they have a sensation when they are about to release the fluid that they are going to urinate so they simply pull it back. They are embarrassed about urinating. Once they are aware of amrita and that they can ejaculate they allow it to happen. If a few drops of urine do come first, what's the problem? The energy circulated by the release of the amrita is far more important than worrying about a little bit of urine. (Be advised that there are current sex videos showing copious quantities of liquid gushing from the woman's vagina. However, the most recent research on this subject by Dr. John Perry shows that, at most, the quantity of female ejaculate released from the G-spot area is no more than the amount of ejaculate released by the male during climax. Therefore, the rest is simply urine.) So when you are pleasuring your partner put down a towel, make it safe for her, and say, "If when I'm pleasuring you you have a sensation of urinating, just go ahead." The urine is a sterile fluid so it can't harm you. However, it can release the amrita and give her a more intense orgasm.

Every woman has the potential to experience the outpouring of this amrita. It doesn't happen every time through any particular technique, although specific techniques that repeatedly stimulate the area of the sacred G-spot are more likely to cause ejaculation. This is not a formula; it happens as a gift.

In tantric writings the amrita is considered to be nutritious. A tiny taste of this can give you a lift in energy. My experience is that this is an incredible energy rush. When the nectar drenches my lingam during lovemaking I feel I've had an energy bath, and that feeling stays with me for days afterward. I find this energy healing and, rejuvenating and a source of enormous power.

In ancient India men returning from battle would go to the temples to have their psychic wounds healed by the high priestesses of love, by these sacred prostitutes or *dakini,* as they were called. Healing with amrita was practiced by these priestesses.

Some women have told Diane and me that they have experienced one-hour extended orgasms and the release of large quantities of amrita—not just drops or spoonfuls as for men, but cupfuls. It may have happened naturally and easily for all women in the golden age of tantra, when the shakti was honored and encouraged, but after more than two thousand years of suppression women's orgasmic energy has been subdued. Awakening a woman's full orgasmic nature is not easy. Men and women have to be taught how to reawaken the shakti.

This process has already begun with women's energy pervading every aspect of our consciousness—scientists are moving more into the study of ecology, which has to do with the feminine principle, the interconnectedness of things, and businesses are being run on different principles—teamwork, networking, and relatedness. Women's groups are studying their goddess nature. It's happening now all around us.

In tantric writings it is said that "tantra is born again from age to age."

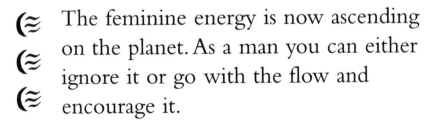 The feminine energy is now ascending on the planet. As a man you can either ignore it or go with the flow and encourage it.

Going against the nature of things is a hard path. If you run your business the old way and want it to work you are heading along a tough path.

What you can do in terms of your lovemaking is to act as a teammate with your partner to awaken the shakti. Once this shakti is awakened it's going to increase your partner's desire; it's going to increase her feeling of pleasure; she is going to want to make love a lot more, and in fact she may become almost insatiable.

On one level you say, "That's great! An insatiable woman," but on another level when you are living with her it can become frightening. The fear is that you might not be able to keep her satisfied. She might look for other men. But as a conscious man you can become a conscious lover through learning the lovemaking secrets. It's time for both lovers to act as teammates in the awakening of the shakti, because when the shakti is flowing it is healing, revitalizing, and rejuvenating for both partners.

Ancient Taoist masters discovered three waters or types of fluid involved in female orgasms. Lubrication experienced during arousal is considered to be the first water. The fluids emitted during normal orgasm are the second water, and the female ejaculation released from the sacred spot is the third water. All three fluids are shakti energy, shakti power, which you can absorb during your lovemaking.

It is a great secret to know that you can benefit from absorbing this shakti, from absorbing the nectar and the love juice. It can energize you and nurture you physically and psychically. The physical uptake happens simply through the natural absorptive capacity of the head of the lingam while you are inside of a woman, hard or soft. The lingam becomes erect by filling with blood. When the lingam becomes soft the membrane naturally absorbs the woman's secretions. Ovarian hormones, minerals, and tissue salts, as well as amino acids and other body-building substances, are some of the highly potent substances contained in yoni juice. Besides the physical absorption you are energetically absorbing her yin essence, psychically absorbing her shakti.

I can't easily describe this type of absorption. It's not a physical substance but you can feel it just by watching your woman having an orgasm; it can charge your energy. Although you haven't physically absorbed anything, you have been psychically charged.

> (≈
> (≈
> (≈
> (≈ **When your woman is orgasming, understand that you are in the presence of shakti power. When that is happening it's very important to drink deeply of that power, absorbing the shakti essence.**

ABSORBING SHAKTI ENERGY

Most men are not aware of the shakti energy, yet it is a subtle energy that you can pick up any time you are in the presence of a woman who is sexually aroused. Men may feel it but they don't know what it is and have no idea how it can benefit them. If you are consciously aware of what shakti energy is, then that consciousness determines how you will use it. If you drink deeply of its energy, you will gain power.

A conscious lover, aware of the power of the shakti energy, will drink deeply of that energy whenever he is in its presence. You should be especially aware at the point of orgasm because the room will fill with this magic energy. Look at your woman. Look how vital and glowing she appears, flushed with the hormones, the energy, the juices that run through her body that can charge and empower you, fill you with creativity and energy. As she orgasms, breathe in deeply and absorb as much of the shakti as you can. Then as you breathe out imagine you are sending the energy back to her.

During orgasm the woman's shakti energy is totally awakened, so use this time to tell her things that support her and her sexuality. Around the time of orgasm the woman is totally open to receiving imprints through the things that you say to her. Never say anything that puts her down or makes her feel bad after orgasm because she is very open then. Utilize this time for healing. Say something about your love for her, how close you feel to her. Or use this as a time to override old patterns that she may have about the shape of her body or her sexual response.

Very often in day-to-day life your partner won't really hear it when you say, "I love your body," "I love your breasts," or "I love the way you look." But in this open psychic state she has no choice. It will sink deeply into her subconscious and she will absorb it. So you can use this as a valuable healing time for your relationship.

This is also a great time to give your partner some positive conditioning in the area of her sexual loving. In ancient India women were taught positive connection with their sexuality. They were taught that with the shakti energy they could create harmony in themselves, in their family, and in the world. Your woman's subconscious may be impregnated with negative experiences, imprints that other men may have given her. Maybe she spent time with a man who never understood her sexually but just pounded away until he ejaculated. This builds up negative imprinting about sexuality, and about men in general. The point of her orgasm provides a great opportunity to heal some of this. In this way you are absorbing the shakti energy and sending energy back to her.

REPLACING ENERGY AFTER EJACULATION

A lot of men in our seminars who have been studying Taoist ejaculation techniques have often taken the application of these too far. They were afraid of ejaculating because they thought they would lose so much lifeforce they would die young. Once they understood they could easily replace that energy with the unlimited power of their partner's love juices it took away a lot of pressure. So if you have ejaculated and you want to replace that energy, make sure the lingam remains in her yoni as long as possible after ejaculation. While you are in there, drink deeply of that essence either through gently "sipping" the love juices by pumping your PC muscle, by imagining you are breathing in her essence, or simply through your consciousness of the power of the shakti, knowing that it can heal you, rejuvenate you, and energize you.

Now that you are aware of shakti power you have another reason for learning ejaculation control. One of the biggest benefits of learning ejaculation control is that, because you are able to be in your beloved's yoni much longer than an average man, you will absorb more shakti from her inexhaustible supply. That essence gives power to your yang essence. Your bond of love presupposes a two-way exchange.

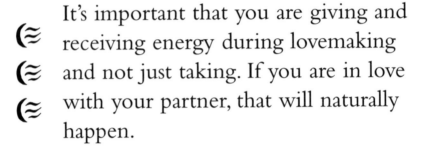

> It's important that you are giving and receiving energy during lovemaking and not just taking. If you are in love with your partner, that will naturally happen.

When you are cycling energy as described in chapter 8 you are giving and receiving energy. Your mouth and genitals are connected and you are mixing nectar but you are also mixing energy, you are actually mixing vital essences and absorbing shakti. There may not be any movement, but you are absorbing each other's essences just by being connected. This same exchange also occurs during karezza. While you are in these positions you can again be thinking of absorbing the shakti and mixing divine essences.

ORAL SEX

Absorption of yoni juices takes place through your mouth as well as the lingam. When you are licking your woman think of it as exchanging vital essences—saliva and yoni juices forming a special nectar to nourish you both. Your thoughts play a vital role in creating a particular energy, so it is important to educate yourself to believe in the benefits of absorbing shakti energy and mixing vital essences. Drink deeply of her love juices; they are healing, rejuvenating, nurturing, vitalizing.

Have this very clearly in your mind when you have lingam in yoni. Think of it as forming a unique elixir that only you two can make. Not only are you bonding together physically and emotionally, but you are mixing your very essences. Science may not yet be able to prove that you are mixing spirits, but I have no doubt that in the future the many levels of energy exchange that occur during lovemaking will be explored and proven as new technology develops. I believe we should not limit our thinking and beliefs to what can be measured; we should rather experiment with thoughts of what might be happening and discover what we experience as a result of those thoughts. This is a much more creative way to approach lovemaking.

Here is another secret for you to try. I suggest that during oral sex (or any lovemaking for that matter) where there is an exchange of sexual juices that contain vital essences, you create a mind-set that you are mixing spirits. Then repeat this belief over and over by imagining that this is happening whenever you are in sexual connect. You will soon get a deep sense of this really happening—that you and your beloved are becoming as one, that your own ego and identity fade away and you become a new energy body. You can take it even further and imagine that new energy body radiating light to nourish and enlighten your own spirit. When you have this attitude your lovemaking, whether genital or oral, becomes a spiritual experience. It has a sense of purity about it and this helps heal any previous negative conditioning you may have picked up. Even though you may be much more open to cunnilingus now because of articles appearing in magazines about how good it is, earlier conditioning can still affect your thoughts while you are giving it. If this ever happens for you or your thoughts are on anything else other than ecstasy, then fill your mind with this new reality and replace those thoughts.

ANOTHER REASON FOR SAYING "YES" TO SEX

The more you make love and the more love juice you absorb, the more closely you will bond because you are sharing vital essences. Imagine you and your lover are linking on a spiritual level. Stay in yoni as long as you can and as much as you can because you are absorbing shakti in the form of energy and nectar. In the soft styles of lovemaking such as karezza, you are absorbing shakti; in Daily Devotion you are absorbing shakti. Every time you are inside a woman you are filling yourself with sexual and spiritual energy.

STAYING YOUNG

During the past twenty years Western society has been obsessed with youth. Staying youthful is a multi-million-dollar business. Men and women who thirty years ago would have retired gracefully to gardening, knitting, reading, relaxing, and looking after the grandchildren are now taking up sports and having operations to remove wrinkles and fat. They want to look young again. We are indoctrinated by the media notion that youth is the only beauty there is. Old is not at all popular. Look at all the advertising—we are bombarded in the media with images of youthful people. Models are popular now at thirteen, but after twenty or so their modeling careers are often in steep decline. The more the desire of our society is to look and feel younger, the more we will devise methods to accomplish it. An article in *New Woman* magazine (1993) stated that

> science is seriously looking at longevity. At Universities and Medical Research Centres around the world the multi-billion-dollar human genome project is under way. Genetic scientists have already isolated genes which cause disease. There is good reason to believe that eventually they will isolate genes that give the body messages to switch itself off—the death genes. They already know the genes of some cancer cells are immortal. Splice together one of these cells with a youthful healthy human cell, snip out one of the cell's forty-six chromosomes—the death chromosomes—and you end up with a healthy immortal human cell.

This breakthrough has been achieved at the National Institutes of Health in the United States and at the Kanagawa Cancer Centre in

Yokohama, Japan. I don't think anything like "immortal cells" will be available commercially in my lifetime, but everyone wants to look and feel young. Probably more important than looking young is feeling young. The study of this in the West is very new. In China longevity has been studied for at least two thousand years. As people grew older in China they were treated with great respect and honor. Ingenious ways were developed to stay in good health in old age because these could be the best years of a person's life.

Many of these ancient methods of keeping youthful have not yet been proven scientifically but they must have worked on some level or they wouldn't have been practiced for two thousand years. The Chinese learned experimentally what worked, and they continued to use and teach these methods. Many people in the West have tried special diets and exercises such as t'ai chi to help them look and feel younger. However, the greatest secret the ancient Chinese discovered for longevity has only recently been made available through the interpretation of ancient texts. Since it's only newly released in the West, it's a fortunate person who has been introduced to this secret.

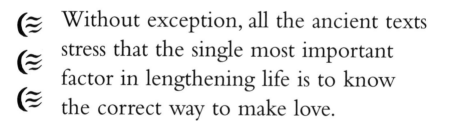 Without exception, all the ancient texts stress that the single most important factor in lengthening life is to know the correct way to make love.

HOW TO LIVE LONGER

Science has established that hormones are closely linked with the aging process, and our sexual machinery includes vital hormone-producing glands. Lovemaking for men in ancient China was concerned primarily with two major aspects. One was the reserving of semen, which I mentioned earlier, and the second was the absorption of women's yoni emissions, physically and psychically. For absorbing this shakti I will give you several practices that promote longevity.

SIPPING

When you have your lingam inside your beloved, sometimes stop all movement and imagine you are gently sipping her love juices through your lingam. You do this by contracting and releasing the PC muscle, the muscle you use to hold back urination. Imagine you are sipping through a straw for one or two minutes.

Obviously you wouldn't do this practice indiscriminately. I strongly advise that you do it with someone you know well. If your beloved has any form of infection you certainly wouldn't use this practice.

It would also be a waste of time practicing this technique while wearing a condom. If you need to use a condom for whatever reason, imagine absorbing the shakti energy psychically rather than physically. Imagine yourself psychically filling up with the shakti power. This can be energizing but nowhere near as powerful as absorbing the actual nectar. This is another good reason for you to work on your relationship—if you don't have to concern yourself with condoms you can freely absorb the vital nectar. It will empower you, rejuvenate and revitalize you. Your woman can similarly sip your juices so you have a mutual exchange occurring.

ABSORBING THE ORGASM

If your woman orgasms, this is a special nectar to absorb. This nectar is very precious, even more precious than normal sexual secretions; it's the most rejuvenating. Take it as a great blessing. Suck up her emissions. Also, if you have ejaculated with her orgasm or after her, the nectar that results from the mixing of your essences is powerful, so take time to absorb as you lie soft inside her.

SLEEP IN YOUR BELOVED

This is a great practice that anyone can do, and it is especially appropriate for busy couples. Lie in the spoon position (on your side with knees bent, your partner enveloped in your arms) or in the scissors position, and slip inside your beloved. Use lubricant if you have to. Try to relax and go to sleep inside her. It's a useful practice when she has come and you do not want to ejaculate that night. If you feel yourself slip out later that is fine, because you know you have absorbed your beloved's nectar. Sometimes you fall asleep while you are still erect and wake up in the morning with a smile on your face because the last thought in your mind before you slept was that you were in yoni. This is great energy to sleep on. The last thoughts you have on your mind before sleep sink deeply into your subconscious and affect you throughout the next day.

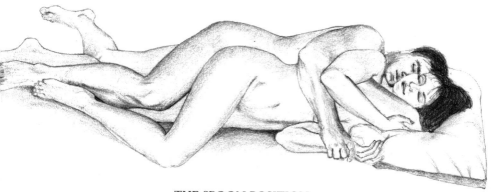

THE SPOON POSITION

MIXING SALIVA AND YONI JUICE

When you are having oral sex the mouth fills with saliva. Mix this saliva with the yoni juice. Think of it forming a special elixir and drink deeply of it. Any repugnance to oral sex is often due to widespread confusion about the difference between bodily excretions, which are waste products no longer needed, and sexual secretions, which are fluids rich in nutrients.

Of course, perfect genital hygiene is a prerequisite for this practice and the sipping practice. If your woman has any form of discharge or any consistent type of vaginal infection, don't use these practices.

Share these practices with your partner only if you feel she is ready. It is a wise lover who doesn't introduce his partner to things before she is ready. If it's going to frighten or turn her off in any way, tell her about them a little bit at a time. In the meantime, you can practice them yourself.

Both tantric and Taoist traditions had many advanced practices for absorption of the woman's essence. These practices were carried out in deep secrecy. In the ancient texts there are many stories of men and women, living well into their hundreds, who practiced absorbing each other's essences. Normally in a healthy relationship any loss of female yin essence is compensated for with absorption of the male yang essence. However, the texts warn that if a man repeatedly forces himself on a woman he may extract her vital energy, or she may drain herself by forcing herself to have sex for the man's benefit or by forcing her orgasm rather than allowing it to occur naturally. Many women force their orgasm to satisfy their man, but it drains their vital essence. If your woman is doing this she will age a lot quicker.

Ancient Chinese and Indian masters clearly understood the power of shakti, and thus would have numerous concubines and wives in order to absorb more shakti to keep young. There are

Hindu rituals in which the man would make love to many women on the one night before implanting his seed into his special number one wife. There are many stories of men living into their hundreds with at least twenty wives—and keeping them all satisfied. These stories were common. Not only did the ancient masters believe that lots of shakti would keep them young, they also believed that it would raise their consciousness and awareness. Thus they kept the secrets from the masses because to the masses they appeared as gods, men of wisdom. This was one of the secrets of their charisma.

You don't need twenty wives to absorb the shakti, because one beloved has all the shakti you can possibly handle. Besides, with the prevalence of sexually transmitted diseases it is not appropriate today to have a lot of lovers.

Your woman's shakti may be suppressed now, but believe me, the potential is unlimited. You need to work as teammates to awaken it. The secret is to realize that for your beloved to open up to that much shakti she really has to trust you. Trust, love, commitment, and practice are all important.

Together you go on this journey. Whenever resistances come up for either you or your beloved, instead of abandoning the relationship work through these problems to reach another level. And always enjoy the journey to opening more shakti—it's unlimited.

 There is always more to your lovemaking. In lovemaking boredom sets in only because you give up exploring.

There is always more love, more openness, more shakti available, and it is available with the woman you are in a relationship with right now. Finding a new woman will raise your excitement level but you will soon come to a point where you can go no further. This is when you need to act as teammates, choosing to maintain love and sexual passion for a lifetime together and agreeing to do whatever is necessary to achieve that. Of course, there are often situations where it's best to move on, but give your relationship every possible chance before doing that.

ACHIEVING THE THINGS YOU WANT

What separates the top 10 percent of men from the rest? hard work? money? power? the people they know? Or is there something else? Yes, frequently there is something else. Lots of yoni! I'm not saying that the other factors aren't powerful in achieving success in life, but very few men know the secret of lots of yoni.

It gives you that leading edge; it gives you that something else. It really does. It empowers you. It gives you a special type of power that other men respect, even though they can't define it. It's like the Mona Lisa—there is something about the smile—and although you can't define it, you still feel it.

I'm not talking about an aggressive power—that power that comes from not getting yoni. The power I am talking about is an inner strength, more like the power of water than that of fire. The world needs more yoni power, more shakti, more of the yin element right now.

If you are in a business and you need that something extra as a manager, then kiss more yoni. You can source the shakti to empower you to achieve whatever you want. The tantric writings say that the god Shiva would be powerless in the phenomenal world without his goddess Shakti. Helping to evoke the shakti by worshiping your woman and loving her and learning all the lovemaking secrets can be a little frightening for some men. You may worry that she will end up taking you over and you won't be able to keep up. "I don't want to make my woman more powerful," you say. In the sixties and seventies, with the women's liberation movement, men were burned; they were over-whelmed by woman's energy, they didn't like it. It was threatening to them. But shakti is not that form of energy. That was a male form of energy. This is the shakti that is more like the water element; it won't burn you. It enhances male and female power. Shakti energy empowers men in the achievement of their personal and business goals.

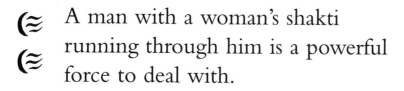 A man with a woman's shakti running through him is a powerful force to deal with.

It makes a world of difference when you have your woman's shakti supporting you. You can tap in to the shakti to empower yourself, and the more that shakti flows the more your beloved is empowered, because the shakti energy is unlimited. The more it flows, the more it generates. It is best to nurture and evoke the shakti lovingly as team-mates; then both of you will be empowered. If either of you force the shakti you may feel drained, even though the shakti is unlimited. Empower your Shakti, your woman, by letting her know she is the source and center of your life. Do not be afraid to give her that recognition. It builds trust.

In one of our workshops, Edward recounted to Diane and me his experience of being empowered by his wife's shakti.

"I've just started a high-powered business. My wife wants to support my new career. She works from home, so often before I'm due at an important meeting I'll call home and ask for some juice for the meeting. She always says yes because that's an agreement we have made. I rush home to Lorraine, I enter her, and we breathe together for ten minutes, just absorbing and sharing the shakti energy, then I go back to work charged for the meeting.

"Her side of the agreement is that we must complete in ten

minutes unless she requests to go on. So when I go back to work I feel really special. It somehow makes me feel great to know my lingam is still covered with juice of my beloved. I know none of the other men in the meeting have just been in yoni and it gives me a lot of confidence as a man."

Elliot, a personal development lecturer in the United States, shared this story with Diane and me.

"Always before a lecture Elishia and I will come into connection and charge each other with energy. In the early stages of my lecturing career I would always be nervous before presenting my lectures in front of a large crowd, so Elishia would always invite me to come and charge up on her shakti energy. I'd take that shakti energy, her sensuality, her sexuality, her juices, and I would be literally covered in them while I was out there giving my lecture.

"I would sit in a chair and Elishia would sit on top of me, pumping away with the shakti energy filling me up with juice and energy. I'd give it back to her by telling her how much I loved her and appreciated the energy and by telling her how she supported me being powerful in the world."

James told us that before he was introduced to the concept of shakti energy being a lifeforce with rejuvenating and healing properties he would engage in oral sex, but usually only to pleasure Jill. He knew that she liked it and he'd often use it as foreplay. But since he has learned the power of drinking Jill's shakti power through her yoni juices, oral sex has become a totally new experience in which he indulges for hours. Oral sex for James now is about rejuvenation, about gaining more power and confidence, and about linking Jill and himself together on a spiritual level.

A lot of people comment to me: "You are a little man, [I'm only 5 feet 8 inches tall] but on stage you appear big. You've got a lot of energy." Little do they know that I'm empowered with shakti, with my beloved's love juices.

10

Jewel Honoring and the G-Spot

This lovemaking secret requires your partner to be in a receiving mode, surrendering to more pleasure than she has ever experienced before, and for you to be in a giving mode, treating her with love, honor, and reverence.

You can start the Jewel Honoring practice with a salutation if you wish, to signify that this is a special lovemaking session. After an appropriate time of foreplay (kissing, stroking, cuddling), when you feel your woman is receptive to you pleasuring her and ready to trust you to serve her, make sure she is in a comfortable position lying on her back and tell her to relax because it's her time to receive. Place a pillow under her head, ask her to rest her arms by her sides and relax her feet so that they're slightly apart. Ask her to allow you to look after her. Make sure the room is warm enough so that she doesn't require heavy covers. You may wish to use a light sheet that you can easily move over her body as you pleasure different areas. Place a towel under her buttocks so she feels safe about releasing ejaculate if that happens to occur.

Start by pleasuring her extremities. On the inside of her arm, make a circular movement tracing an oval shape between the wrist and the elbow to make the biggest oval possible. If one fingertip is too ticklish for her, use all your fingers or the flat of your hand and firm pressure. As you trace out this shape keep your mind in the moment, focusing on the pleasure you are feeling in your fingertips as well as the pleasure you sense she might be feeling. Be sensitive and conscious of what you are doing. Let your focus be on pleasure; get some feedback from her as to whether she would like your touch to be softer, firmer, slower, or faster. Every time she responds say, "Thank you!" If she requests a firmer stroke, then increase the firmness and ask, "Firmer still?"

Good communication is vital. First, it keeps you and your partner present and focused on what you are doing. Second, you may think you know what your partner likes but you are not a mind reader, so it's best to ask. Third, it is sometimes difficult for a woman to say what she wants during sex, so this gives her the opportunity to lead you to what gives her the most pleasure. As I have said before, a great secret of lovemaking is to give your partner more of what she wants rather than what you think she wants. Fourth, because she is in this position of surrendering to pleasure she can feel quite vulnerable, so your communication allows her to trust you more because she knows what to expect.

Don't do unexpected things, such as suddenly putting your hand on her yoni when she is in this vulnerable position. That can break her trust and direct her thoughts to what you are going to do next rather than her being in the present moment and enjoying the pleasure. Men feel they should automatically know how to stimulate a woman so they often don't ask, and women are often afraid to say because they don't want to bruise their man's ego. So a woman often goes on silently enduring ineffectual stimulation. In an earlier chapter I outlined how to tell your partner what you want in a nonblaming way. This nonblaming communication is important to follow in this practice of Jewel Honoring.

As you proceed with pleasuring your partner's lower arm, keep communicating as you make the oval smaller and smaller, spiraling in as you go toward a center point. Finally, place your fingers steadily on the center point and stop for a few seconds. Trace similar circles around sensitive areas, such as the inside of the wrist and the inside of the elbow.

This type of stimulation builds up the energy in the body to a state of intensity that we call tumescence. There's a lot of pleasure in tumescence, but a woman reaches a point where she needs to be de-tumesced. This is done by stopping all movement or by using firm pressure, which creates another form of pleasure. So after you've stopped at a center point, de-tumesce the whole lower part of the arm using a long, firm stroke with the flat of your palm, continuing to stroke from the inside of the elbow right out through her hand and fingertips. Then move to the upper part of her arm and continue the same process of stimulating the area with the concentric circles coming in toward the center. Finish by de-tumescing the whole arm with a long, firm stroke.

Remember to check in with her. Kiss her, stroke her hair and face, tell her that you love her, that you love pleasuring her, so that she feels safe and loved and doesn't feel like an object. Then move to the other arm and do the same circular pleasuring process. Do the same with her breasts, moving from bigger to smaller circles as you get to the center point. Then brush lightly across the nipple in a teasing manner before you touch it. Eventually touch the nipple with sensitivity, with awareness, holding steady. Then wet your fingertips with saliva and gently roll the nipple with your fingertips. Some women don't like their breasts being touched too much, especially if they have just been breast-feeding an infant, so before you touch this area ask her if it's okay. When tumescence has built up in the breasts and the nipples are erect, de-tumesce the breasts by cupping them in your hands and gently but firmly rotating the breasts in circles. You can do both breasts at once after you have tumesced and de-tumesced them individually.

Now move to your partner's legs. To reach the inside of the leg, gently bend her leg at the knee and place it on a pillow to the side. Pleasure one leg, then the other. All this time her yoni could be covered with a sheet or a sarong. It's nice to use a light cover the first few times you do this practice, especially if you're with a relatively new partner.

Spend ten to fifteen minutes on the whole body before you take your attention to your woman's yoni. Many of you will have had your attention on the yoni most of the time you were pleasuring the whole body, but you must learn to keep your mind on what you are doing at the present moment—then the whole experience can be pleasure and not just the goal at the end. Once you've pleasured the rest of your woman's body place your hand gently over her yoni, cupping the whole area. Place your other hand on her heart center. Again, remember to kiss her and show her you care for her.

Now carefully apply lubricant to your partner's whole genital area, inside the labia, starting from the base of the yoni and moving up the insides toward and around the clitoral area while being careful to only gently brush this area. Just as you did with the rest of the body, start the circular motions, being careful to avoid the clitoris. This is the last point you touch, the point of most pleasure, so you build up the energy before you touch the clitoris. Move very slowly, making your circles for several minutes before you eventually circle around the clitoris. As you get closer

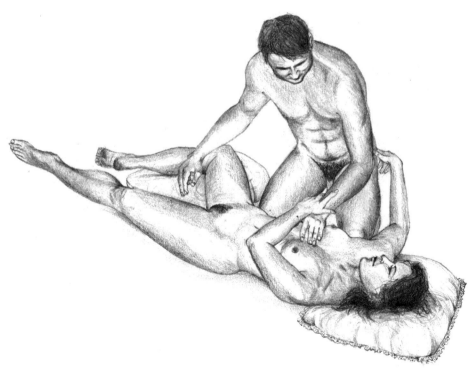

HONORING THE JEWEL

only gently brush across the clitoral area, almost like teasing it.

The clitoris is the jewel. The clitoris has no other purpose than to give a woman pleasure. At this point in your Jewel Honoring process your woman has totally surrendered to allowing you to give her pleasure. Once you get to the jewel, stay there. Don't keep moving back all over her body again. Start to pleasure the jewel and surrounding area by finding a stroke that your partner likes. Try different areas and different pressures. Sometimes it's more sensitive on the left, sometimes on the right. Some women don't want it touched directly at all and what feels good today doesn't always feel the same the next day. What feels good at the beginning often changes toward the end of a session.

Unfortunately, there is no reliable formula; each woman is unique and each time it is different. This is why communication is vital. Ask your woman how she would like to be touched. Asking her these questions seems silly at first but you will soon get over that. It's a great pleasure to know you are doing it just right and she is getting more of what she wants. Don't change from one stroke to another too quickly; give her time to relax with the stroke and to see how it feels. Once you find a stroke your partner likes, continue with a consistent stroke. Women hate it when you are doing well and then you change your movement.

As a general rule, make your strokes slow, reliable, and steady. Watch your partner's response. What normally happens after a while is that the particular area that is giving a lot of pleasure doesn't feel as pleasurable as it did initially, and you will see this in her response. So gradually change your stroke or experiment by moving to another area. As you continue and she moves into higher states of pleasure, the communication becomes much less frequent. Asking for directions when she is in a highly aroused state can be distracting. In the earlier stages, as you are finding the particular strokes and her particular areas, you ask questions, but as she moves through that use less questioning.

You will eventually get to know your partner's responses much better after you have practiced this for quite some time. But in the early stages when you are not as aware of your partner's response look for signs of arousal—swelling of the yoni, lots of yoni juice, sexual sounds, movement of her pelvis toward your hand, and curling of the toes and feet. Once you see this happening you know you are on the right track.

As she builds toward a peak, where the yoni is very engorged, stop and hold your fingers gently over the clitoral area. This de-tumesces the energy so the pleasure can spread throughout her whole body. Then gently start the stroking again, perhaps in a new area. If you happen to find a very sensitive area at this stage just stroke it a couple of times, then leave it. Keep it for when you wish to take her to orgasm. Peak her several times like this, where she builds up to a heightened, excited state—fully engorged—then hold the area and de-tumesce. Repeat the stroke to build tumescence again and then de-tumesce. Eventually, as she's very close to orgasm, move back to that very sensitive point that you found before and take her right through to orgasm with that point. Once she has orgasmed it is not the end of her pleasure, as she has the potential to orgasm again.

After kissing and cuddling for a few moments, go back to the yoni and ever so gently begin to stimulate the jewel area again. Use lots of lubricant, such as a petroleum-based jelly, rather than a thin oil, because at this stage her jewel is very sensitive to touch directly. You might need to start with only blowing on the jewel. Eventually your partner will begin to respond again and you can go on to a second, third, or fourth orgasm, or even more.

Of course this won't happen for most women the first time you do your honoring; however, with practice, with your partner trusting you more and with your increasing expertise, you will eventually develop a lovemaking skill that you will treasure for a lifetime. Jewel Honoring is one of the most powerful lovemaking secrets you can know.

The benefits of mastering Jewel Honoring are many.

- You have a way of making love that enables you to give a woman pleasure whenever she wants it. Your self-image skyrockets when you know you have this ability.
- You will be able to make love in this way at any age. You don't have to get an erection.

- If your partner's sex drive is stronger than yours it's no longer a problem for you.
- If you ejaculate too soon, you have a way to continue pleasuring your woman until she climaxes.
- If you feel you might come too soon during intercourse you can stop and move into Jewel Honoring. Honor her first until she comes, then continue with intercourse. If you've honored her very well she will be so fully satisfied she won't care if you come quickly. Any performance pressure you may have been feeling is removed.
- Some men don't like making love when their partner is menstruating. With Jewel Honoring this is no longer a problem; you can make love all through the month. Another advantage is that if a man is not having intercourse due to menstruation he tends to touch his partner less often, and this can create problems for a couple that they may not even be aware of. Once you practice Jewel Honoring and you are making love all through the month, you will see the difference in your relationship. You will both be much easier to live with during this sometimes difficult time of the month.
- It's a great way to de-tumesce your partner. If you have noticed her starting to get uptight it may be time to give her a hug and offer her a pleasure session. She might resist at first, but she will bless you afterward.
- Although contact with the hand isn't 100 percent safe in terms of disease transmission, it's a thousand times safer than genital contact. Jewel Honoring should be part of every young person's education on nonpenetrative sex.

Once you become a master of this technique you will never fear that your woman will leave you. No one will be able to get her as high as you can. She will find pleasures beyond anything she has ever imagined because with this technique she learns to fully receive. She learns to trust you to look after her so she can totally surrender her pleasure. You will be able to take her even higher than she can take herself, because when she is pleasuring herself she will resist at certain points. When you are doing it you'll be able to nurture her through those points of resistance. Once she trusts you enough, she will allow you to take her to places of higher pleasure than she has ever experienced.

I know that after reading this chapter many men will say, "I already do this; I play with her yoni!" It's great that you do, but don't be mistaken—this Jewel Honoring practice is far more than playing around with your woman's vagina or stroking her clitoris as foreplay. This is a main event in itself. Once you practice it you will see the difference.

Don't treat this technique lightly. A very similar technique has been experimented with at More University in the United States, and of all the techniques tried during more than twenty years of research there, it is the one that has taken women to the highest states of orgasm—the most pleasurable, the longest, and the most intense. If you don't see a difference between what you normally do and this, then do the process step-by-step and you soon will. It may raise issues and resistances that relate to your partner having enough trust in your expertise to allow herself to go totally out of control. If you can work through these issues and not give up, your relationship will never be the same again!

RESISTANCES

I discussed resistances to pleasure in an earlier chapter and I want to elaborate because, of all the techniques we have shared with people, Jewel Honoring brings up the most resistances for most people. That doesn't mean you should avoid trying it. In fact, quite the opposite— working through these resistances gives you the opportunities to develop deeper love and more trust and allows you to receive and experience higher states of sexual pleasure than you allow yourself now.

Everyone has sexual resistances on some level. If you didn't then you would probably forget to eat and everyone would have extended orgasms every time they made love. Some of these resistances are conscious, but most are subconscious, developed from past conditioning, religious prohibitions, parents' rigid attitudes, and negative experiences. This is especially true for women. Resistances block feelings—the neurotransmitters from the genitals to the brain get blocked. It's been shown that a woman can physically experience vaginal contractions, which sexual researchers would call orgasm, yet at the same time it is not being recorded in her brain as pleasure.

By using Jewel Honoring to work through resistances to reach higher states of pleasure some of these blocked channels can be cleared. As new channels are formed your woman begins to experience much stronger orgasm. Pleasure signals move more quickly and clearly to her brain, enabling her to orgasm more easily and more deeply. These resistances often show up as thoughts. While you are honoring her jewel, she might be thinking, "I don't want to do this!" "This is silly!" "He's just using me!" "I'm not going to be able to orgasm!" "This isn't pleasure!" or "He's not doing it right!"

And you might be thinking, "She's not responding!" "I can't do this, this doesn't work!" "I wish she would come!" "She's bossing me around!" These thoughts are normal, but to make sure you don't entertain them try replacing them with other, positive thoughts. One that Diane and I love to use is "I am loved and I love you." Just keep repeating that to yourself as these negative thoughts cross your mind. Another thing you can try when these thoughts appear is to take your focus to the breath and PC-muscle contractions. Breathe out aloud— "Aahhh"—and in deeply so your partner hears you, and ask her to breathe with you. Tell her beforehand, that if she wants to stay more focused on her pleasure, to use her breath and PC-muscle contractions throughout the pleasuring whenever her mind drifts away from the pleasure.

Besides thoughts, resistances may also show up for your woman as loss of feeling in the yoni. She will show less engorgement, she may pull away, or she may open her eyes and look bored. When this happens men usually stroke harder and faster, but this rarely works. It is better to go much slower and lighter or stop altogether. Ask her what she wants, tell her you love her, and give her some attention. It is a big breakthrough for a woman to be able to totally surrender, to let you look after her pleasure, to allow you to take control. What she is surrendering to is more pleasure for herself, but in going to new places fear often arises, so she needs to be able to trust you.

You need to do whatever is necessary to give your woman enough trust in you to let her shakti go—to release her orgasms to you. This is a great opportunity for you to look at your relationship with your partner and make it more secure. Give her reason to have trust in you. Let her know your love is true and reliable in all circumstances and you will always be there for her.

You can give your partner even more reason to trust you by developing confidence in your ability as a lover. Become a masterful artist with your hands and heart so she can feel the love and confidence in every stroke. Allow her to direct you to her most pleasurable areas and surrender to letting her be your teacher in bed. This is difficult for many men, but if you do this your reward will be learning how to take your partner to a state of pleasure higher than she has ever experienced before.

Tom and Eva had been living together for four years. Eva wanted to get married, but Tom was always putting it off. They didn't have any children; they had a good sex life and made love a lot. When we introduced Jewel Honoring to them they were anxious to try it. Even though Tom often made love to Eva orally and with his hands, they wanted to try the exact Jewel Honoring technique.

The next time we saw them I asked them how it was.

Tom said it was a disaster. He said that it had started off okay. "She liked the body pleasuring and she liked me stroking her jewel. After about fifteen minutes she was really engorged but no matter how much I tried she couldn't orgasm. I peaked her about five times, then she started criticizing what I was doing and getting very angry. After an hour she ended up crossing her legs, pushing me away, and telling me to leave her alone. I eventually pacified her and we started to have intercourse. However, because I had been pleasuring her for over an hour and had watched her yoni engorging, I was tense because she wasn't coming. As soon as I entered her I ejaculated after only a few strokes. I was upset! Eva was upset! She turned her back, brought herself to orgasm, and I was left feeling terrible!"

I told Tom and Eva to try not to worry about it. It is not uncommon for people to have difficulty the first few times. Think of it this way: the first time you make love it isn't always what you expect it to be.

I suggest that the first time you try Jewel Honoring don't think about orgasm; just focus on how much pleasure you are giving and receiving. It's a pleasure being touched, it's a pleasure having undivided attention for one hour, it's a pleasure touching your beloved's yoni, it's a pleasure having the jewel stroked, it's a pleasure stroking the jewel, it's a pleasure looking at the yoni for one hour. It's all pleasure, but too often the mind focuses on a destination and misses the journey. If you focus on pleasure you can't lose. Put your attention on pleasure, not production; that's the secret.

I advised Tom and Eva to do the Jewel Honoring process for only fifteen minutes next time, noting how much they could keep their minds on pleasure. I suggested they have a break during which they acknowledge their mutual pleasure, then go on with something else or perhaps make love in their normal ways. I also told Tom that while he is pleasuring Eva's body to try to stay mentally with that pleasure, rather than thinking about where it is leading.

STAY IN THE MOMENT

When stroking the jewel be totally tuned in to what you are doing. This is a good skill for men to develop in any lovemaking session to keep their mind on the moment, not the sensation at the end—the ejaculation, or the woman's orgasm. A great tantric teacher, Osho, once said: "Keep your attention on the fire at the beginning and stay with that, rather than focus on the embers at the end." Having your mind rush ahead to the orgasm makes you too hot by the time you enter. That is why Tom came so quickly. Keep your mind on the pleasure of the moment.

The next time Tom and Eva tried this practice things went much better. They practiced several times in the manner I had suggested, gradually extending the time. After six months Eva managed to orgasm while Tom was pleasuring her. During these six months they were also making love in their usual ways. But Jewel Honoring was a breakthrough for them because the only way Eva had orgasmed previously was by stroking her own jewel while Tom was inside or when he gave her oral sex. Now she was orgasming much more easily and strongly than ever before—and Tom was creating it.

I told them the process is very powerful and may continue to bring up occasional resistances, but the rewards outweigh the burdens. As the resistances clear the orgasms get better. I reminded Tom that Jewel Honoring has to do with trust and that it might be even better once they were married because Eva would trust enough to go further into her shakti with him. One year later they married and Jewel Honoring is now one of their normal ways of making love, as it is for many other couples to whom Diane and I have introduced this technique.

HELPFUL TIPS FOR JEWEL HONORING

LUBRICATION

Remember that the jewel itself doesn't produce natural secretions like the yoni does, so use plenty of lubrication. For some people oil or KY Jelly makes the jewel too sensitive to stroke. If this is happening I suggest you use petroleum jelly. A lubricant of this consistency works much better for Jewel Honoring, especially when you reach the stage of extended pleasuring into multiple orgasms, where there can be a lot of stimulation of the jewel over a long time.

STROKES YOU USE

If you are not sure what strokes to use to give your woman maximum pleasure, then ask her if you may watch her pleasuring herself and learn what she does. Another great way to learn is to have her take your fingers and pleasure herself with your hand. Keep your fingers very soft and flexible and give over control to her.

Some women actually get little pleasure from stimulation of the clitoris because they have turned off to clitoral response altogether. This is sometimes due to negative conditioning from parents about masturbation. These women are not able to respond sensually with clitoral stimulation alone; they respond only to deep penetration. They might feel guilty about experiencing pleasure any other way, so very early in their lives their minds turned off to self-stimulation.

It's no good pushing a woman by continuing to stroke, as she won't respond no matter what stroke you use. She needs to open much more to her own sexuality. It could be helpful for her to study and practice women's self-pleasuring secrets and perhaps consult a sex therapist. Encourage her to do this because it's a pity to miss out on Jewel Honoring. It's a great way to open your woman to multiple orgasms, so it is something worth including in your lovemaking.

FINDING THE JEWEL

The size and shape of the jewel varies considerably from woman to woman. With some women it's easy to find; however, with most you need to pull back the lips of the yoni with the fingers of one hand while you stroke the jewel with the other. If you have any difficulty your woman can pull back the lips herself by placing two hands above the pubic bone to expose the jewel. It would be good to do this the first few times you try Jewel Honoring.

CHECKING IN WITH YOUR PARTNER

Give your partner loving attention and make her feel special. Ask her permission before you even touch her sacred place. This helps her feel special and safe in your hands.

A lot of women say that during this practice they often feel like an object because their man is so intently focusing only on the yoni, only on her orgasm, and that he doesn't give enough attention to her. To avoid this stop the stroking several times, stop the stroking altogether; talk; kiss; look in to her eyes and remind her that you love her. Also tell her what is going on. Give her feedback. She can't see her own yoni, so tell her how beautiful she looks. Tell her about the lovely shape and color of her yoni; tell her her yoni is like a beautiful flower opening; tell her how her labia are engorging. Tell her how much you enjoy her and how marvelous you feel being able to pleasure her.

KEEP COMMUNICATING

One woman said that when her partner asked her if she wanted the stimulation to the left or right or faster or slower she wasn't sure so she couldn't answer. Diane advised her: "It's best to answer in any way to maintain communication. Otherwise he doesn't know what is going on, whether he is doing it correctly or not. Simply say, 'To the left!' If you find that doesn't give you any more pleasure, still say "thank you," then ask him to move a little to the right or up or down or to somewhere else, until he finds a sensitive spot for you. Every time you give him a direction and he follows it, remember to thank him so you stay in communication."

I have said many times before that it's not just technique that results in good sex. Your partner is not a machine that responds by pressing certain buttons and following manuals step-by-step and I don't want you to think of Jewel Honoring like that. At the same time it is a technique that every great lover should know.

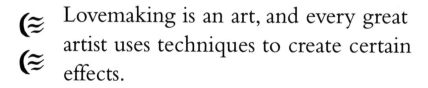 Lovemaking is an art, and every great artist uses techniques to create certain effects.

There are many techniques. Some, as explained in this book, bring more heart and emotion into your lovemaking. Others help you to make your lovemaking a spiritual experience. Jewel Honoring provides a way to explore just how much physical sexual pleasure you can give your partner.

It's often a good practice to take these three areas of lovemaking separately—the emotional, the spiritual, and the physical—and take time to develop each one. You can say to yourself, "This week I'm going to practice feeling more love while having sex." To do that you might use more of the soft sex styles, such as karezza. Another time you may choose to use your lovemaking as a meditation or a devotion. Another week you might explore how much sexual pleasure you can give your partner, or how many orgasms she can have in one session. Then all of these aspects combine and start to come alive in your everyday lovemaking; they become intertwined. Jewel Honoring is a technique to create more physical sexual pleasure for your woman, but at the same time you are touching her with love. You can regularly communicate to her your love. You can use the experience as a meditation, putting your mind and body and heart into every touch. Everything you do during Jewel Honoring can be done with reverence, creating a sacred experience.

Ideally you would not need to practice any of these skills or learn any of these sexual secrets. Sex should just happen naturally—just as love and life should happen smoothly and naturally. But unfortunately that is not the case. We will always be developing more life skills. Love and sex are a big part of life and, like anything else, should be studied and practiced so we improve them. Our children will be better off if we do because there is a chance for them to get a healthy upbringing in the area of lovemaking. Sex and love are the strongest energy transmitters we experience in our bodies, so there is always going to be more for us to explore and develop in these areas.

I've devoted a lot of space to this chapter because I believe Jewel Honoring provides a lifetime of unlimited potential for you to explore sexual love and passion. With practice you will get better at the technique, but you will reach a stage where you will not be able to get your woman any higher until she trusts you more. At that point you will need to open more and more to your love and you will need to commit yourself totally to your beloved so that she feels safe. She needs to know that you deeply love her and you will always be there for her. Only then will she let go into deeper multiple orgasms with you. You might think, "No matter how good my technique, no matter how much I love her, she will have to educate and develop herself more in love, in her sexuality, and that's up to her." True enough, she will need to develop herself and work on herself as you are doing. There are excellent books and women's groups available to assist her. However, you can facilitate that awakening better than any group or book or therapist with your love and your consciousness, because you are the only one who she allows to touch her sexually. The greatest healing can happen when your woman is physically experiencing more love and sexual pleasure. No book can do that for her.

You are potentially your partner's greatest sexual healer, as she is yours.

AWAKENING THE G-SPOT

As with Jewel Honoring, this is a technique that honors sexual pleasure but at the same time you bring in your open-heartedness, your love, and your consciousness about using lovemaking as a sacrament.

Most of you will have heard about the G-spot so I will concentrate on teaching you how to awaken it for your partner. The G-spot was after by a German gynecologist, Dr. Grafenberg.

A book called *The G-spot,* published in 1982, described the location of this erogenous area. However, at the time there was little understanding of how this spot functioned and a lack of knowledge about how to awaken it. Once the media got hold of the information, men received the impression that simply stimulating the G-spot would bring a woman to orgasm. Men began searching around the yoni, looking for this magic button. In most cases they were disappointed. Often a man would refer to a drawing of a vagina in a book, then literally poke around looking for the G-spot. After about five minutes of this his partner would start to feel like an object and get annoyed. He would get frustrated because he couldn't find it or couldn't get her to feel any pleasure, and they would end up in conflict. Many men and women gave up looking for the G-spot.

There has been much written and talked about the G-spot in the past ten years, but we find that our clients, even though they may have experimented from time to time, usually after reading an article still haven't experienced all that they thought might happen. Mostly this is because they haven't persisted for long enough or didn't have the best knowledge and practices of the art of awakening this sacred part of a woman's body.

I hope the sexual secrets I offer here will change all that, because there is so much potential contained in this area for expanding a woman's sexual pleasure, for healing past insecurities and guilt or negative residue attached to her sexuality, for her to move from one orgasm to many orgasms in the one session, and for her to experience deeper, longer, and more intense orgasms than she does now.

The G-spot was not discovered by Dr. Grafenberg. Ancient tantric writings offer much information on the existence of this area. Many tantric teachers refer to this area as a sacred spot. They say the clitoris and the G-spot are like the North and South Poles of the woman's pleasure center, the yang and the yin of the second energy center, the sexual chakra. The location of this sacred spot varies considerably from woman to woman. Sometimes it's deeply set inside the yoni (about 2.75–4 inches) on the upper wall behind the pubic bone. For others it is only about 1 inch inside the vagina. The area feels ridged and the spot often swells during sexual arousal. It can feel like a small pea under your finger; sometimes the spot is much larger.

To give a woman pleasure through the sacred spot, don't poke around the yoni looking for a button; instead, stroke the whole sacred spot area. Only stimulate the area after the woman has been highly sexually aroused, or perhaps after she has already had an orgasm. Most women don't get much pleasure from this area unless there is already a high degree of sexual arousal, and that's why premature searching around for the G-spot doesn't work.

The first time you try to awaken the G-spot I strongly suggest you see this as a pleasuring session rather than an orgasmic session. Orient your thoughts and intention toward pleasure, loving, healing, and awakening of the sacred spot rather than toward orgasm and performance goals. Once you can do this successfully and your woman is highly charged by your stroking of the sacred spot area, then you can explore its orgasmic potential.

PLEASURING YOUR PARTNER
THROUGH THE G-SPOT

Before the session make sure you have plenty of pillows around to get yourselves into comfortable positions, so you have access to your partner's jewel with one hand and her yoni with the other. I like using my left hand for stroking the jewel and my right hand for stimulating the sacred spot, but you should use whatever position you find comfortable.

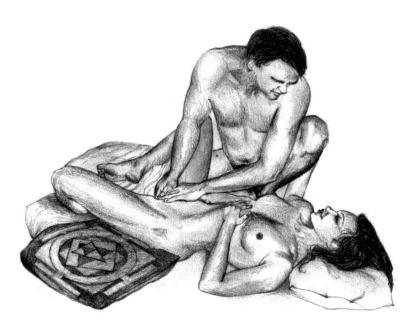

JEWEL AND THE G-SPOT CONNECTION

If you have been Jewel Honoring then your beloved is already in a good position.

It's a good idea to put a towel underneath your partner. Have lubricant nearby. You will need to use lots of lubricant for this whether your partner is naturally lubricated or not. A water-based lubricant is the best. Make sure the room is warm and that she has emptied her bladder before a sacred-spot session.

To start the session, first massage and arouse your partner in whatever ways turn her on before attempting to touch the sacred spot area. You could start with Jewel Honoring and use this practice as an extension of that, or incorporate it as part of lovemaking during intercourse. It is especially useful in situations when your woman is highly aroused but you feel you can't go on, either because you can't hold your ejaculation any longer or because you are losing your erection. Then you could stop intercourse and start to pleasure your woman in this way. Whatever the case, before entering the yoni and reaching for the sacred-spot area make sure she is fully aroused. Her vaginal lips and jewel should be engorged and there should be lots of vaginal secretion.

Once she has reached this stage of sexual excitement, put one hand over her yoni and one on her heart. Kiss her, affirm your love, and make eye contact. Let her see and feel your love. Ask her if you may enter her yoni, her sacred space, and think of it as a great blessing to enter her temple. Asking her in this way will make you both feel special.

Make sure there is lots of lubricant on your hands and fingers. Gently enter the yoni with the ring and forefinger joined together, rather than the index finger, which is more rigid and less flexible than the other two. Take them fully into the yoni. To reach the sacred spot you need to curl your fingers up to touch the upper wall of the yoni in a twelve o'clock position and the pressure needs to be quite firm. Increase the pressure slowly and gradually. Watch her response to the pressure and hold this position for a moment to let her get used to the feeling, then start to pull the fingers toward you along the top of the yoni wall to the front of the yoni, all the way to the pubic bone, in a beckoning type of motion. This completes one stroke.

As you continue to stroke affirm to your woman that you like doing this with her. Continue to stroke in a rhythmic, reliable, steady manner, only one or two strokes per second. Most men have a tendency to move harder and faster in response to their woman's arousal, or they become more active thinking she will respond more. However, judging by the feedback from hundreds of women this isn't always the case. In fact, more often stimulation that is too hard or too fast is a turn-off. Start slowly to let her assimilate the feeling. Don't expect responses, just enjoy being inside your partner. Be aware of your breathing—use your breath-release, muscle-release, and thought-release skills. Breathe aloud, making a sound on the out-breath—"Aahhh"—to encourage her to breathe also. Ask her to breathe with you if you feel she is showing any signs of resistance.

I'll suggest a sequence and timing for the strokes, but as you practice together many times you will get to know which rhythm to use and when. To begin with, start with ten- to twenty-stroke cycles, stop for a second, relax, and then start another cycle of ten to twenty strokes. Repeat this for three or four cycles. Try a couple of cycles in the eleven o'clock position instead of twelve o'clock (where you are stroking now). Watch her response to see what gives her the most pleasure. Many women may not respond immediately to the G-spot stimulation because their pleasure is normally associated with stimulation of the jewel. In these situations you need to make a connection between the G-spot, the jewel, and pleasure.

THE SECRET OF JEWEL–G-SPOT CONNECTIONS

Once you have stimulated your woman through the G-spot, leave the fingers of one hand in the yoni and with your other hand begin to stimulate the jewel area, which was awakened before you entered. If engorgement isn't strong your woman will soon start to respond again, because most women strongly associate the clitoris with pleasure. Through the clitoris bring her into a high pleasure state again, then hold the fingers of the other hand still on the jewel area and go back to the sacred spot, stroking again for a couple of cycles, then go back to the jewel stimulation again. Alternate between the jewel and the sacred spot three or four times. Then stroke the jewel and invite your beloved to pleasure herself while you are stroking inside. The neurotransmitters to the brain have pleasure and jewel associations. You are making G-spot and jewel associations, so that eventually she gets G-spot and pleasure associations.

Remember, in this session your focus is on pleasure, not orgasm. If orgasm occurs that's okay, but orgasm is not the goal. To complete the session, stop and again hold her yoni and her heart. Tell your beloved how much you enjoyed pleasuring her. Move the sexual energy into your heart and feel your love as much as possible. You could sit up in yab-yum and do some cycling of energy together.

It would be best if you didn't go on to intercourse the first time you do sacred-spot work, because if the intercourse doesn't happen the way you expect you might tend to associate that "bad" experience with the sacred-spot work. You want to associate the sacred spot with pleasure, so it's best to leave it at that. This whole process of the sacred-spot pleasuring session connecting with the clitoris should only go on for about ten to fifteen minutes the first time you try it.

Of course, if you have a way of ensuring that your woman will always come, then completing the session with an orgasm could be fine. Otherwise, suggest to your partner that you feel so good and charged and so much in love that you would like to take this energy out to dinner with her. Make the whole night a lovemaking session. You can make love again when you come home. If she is still too charged, lie her down and give her a firm massage. Spread the energy throughout her whole body with long firm strokes. Tell her you are spreading all the shakti she has generated throughout her body for health, vitality, youth, and beauty. Have her visualize herself full of life, vigor, health, love, and vitality.

Engage in several pleasuring sessions like this until you both feel comfortable with doing the sacred-spot work. Don't give up when you encounter resistances, but instead work through them together. If she is not getting much pleasure out of it, don't make her feel bad by trying to push her further each time. Just include the sacred-spot massage as part of your normal lovemaking, as you do with kissing her breasts, perhaps. Try it for just five minutes in a lovemaking session. For some women it may take months before their sacred spot awakens.

Once your woman has had several positive experiences of sacred-spot pleasuring you can add some or all of the following to create even more pleasure.

- During the beckoning stroke, as you draw your fingers toward the pubic bone you will find an area more textured and coarser than the back of the yoni. Hold steady on this area or any area you perceive as giving her more pleasure than the rest.
- Sweep your fingers left and right of center by rotating your wrist, forming a crescent-shaped movement across the sacred spot.
- Tap the sacred-spot area to create a pulsing sensation so your whole hand beats like a pulse as you tap.
- Stimulate the jewel with your left hand while you vibrate the G-spot with the fingers of your other hand.

Remember to stop regularly to allow the energy to spread. The pauses are very powerful. Continual movement often becomes too intense, so stopping allows her to integrate the pleasure. Pause and be still. Timing is important. If you continue to move too quickly and for too long without a pause, you can short-circuit the energy buildup your partner is experiencing. When the sensation is too strong for a beginner to integrate she shuts down altogether; a resistance comes up and that resistance can manifest as decreased sensation, irritability, or an emotional outburst, or your partner may tense her body and hold her breath. If this happens stop, breathe deeply, and withdraw if necessary. Touch her heart, connect with her eyes, send her your love, hold her tightly. Then after a while ask her if she would like you to continue or if she has any requests.

If you connect the sacred spot enough times with pleasure, eventually the mind gets the connection. It is a great secret to know how to make sexual-pleasure connections within the body and mind. It is said that there is a connection between the nipples and the uterus and some say that there is a physical connection between the clitoris and the G-spot, that the roots of the clitoris extend up into the G-spot area. Whether this is true or not, what we are doing is energetically connecting these areas, connecting them in the mind, so that whenever the G-spot is touched it is associated with pleasure.

One of our clients told Diane and me that the first time her boyfriend tried this technique with her she went into an altered state of consciousness for two days afterward. Jenny couldn't believe she could feel so good and she fell deeply in love with Wayne all over again.

Wayne and Jenny had been together for eight months, and, although Wayne had stimulated Jenny with his hand before, it was usually only in foreplay in order to excite her enough for intercourse. This time he had spent twenty minutes just using his hands. He said he couldn't believe how excited she became and how excited it made him feel watching her yoni engorge and pulsate the way it did, her whole body jerking at times.

He said, "I know you said to stop and leave it at that, but there was no way I could possibly stop there. I wanted to enter her so badly but I was so charged from doing this with Jenny and watching her, I thought that if I entered I might not be able to hold my ejaculation. So instead I brought her to orgasm with my mouth, then entered and came myself."

What Wayne did was great and it's common for men, the first time they do this with a woman who responds like Jenny, to not be able to hold that amount of pleasure. However as you make love in this way many times you learn to integrate the pleasure a lot more. It's like when you have intercourse for the first time—it's a lot to handle. I told Wayne to try deep breathing while pleasuring Jenny this way to shift the energy up to his heart, and to make more eye contact with Jenny.

Men very often get too intense the first time they do this pleasuring. They focus totally on the yoni and get mesmerized, then they can't hold that amount of pleasure and at the end of the session they try to enter, only to ejaculate in a few strokes. They get disappointed because they haven't been able to satisfy their woman the way they would have liked to.

Ron and Cassandra are a highly motivated, successful couple who have been married for five years. They did a workshop with Diane and me in 1989. We introduced them to Jewel Honoring. When we saw them again about two years later they told us that they were using Jewel Honoring consistently with their lovemaking. They had to work through some resistances in the earlier stages but now Cassandra was orgasming 90 percent of the time with Ron using Jewel Honoring on its own. So when we introduced them to G-spot pleasuring they were quite anxious to try it and didn't expect any problems.

However, this was not the case. Cassandra didn't feel any pleasure at all in the sacred-spot area. All she felt was burning and a feeling that she wanted to urinate, even though she had been to the toilet several times. When stimulated the sacred-spot area can press on the bladder and create this feeling of wanting to urinate. However, it's only the feeling the mind associates with urination rather than a physical need to urinate. I told her that if she could relax through that feeling it would pass, and that if she was concerned she could put several towels under her and allow it to happen. Most likely she'll find nothing will happen so she can relax and let go of the fear that she might urinate. Once the fear passes the feeling very often transforms into pleasure.

The burning sensation Cassandra experienced is very common. Some women experience areas of pain also, and this I feel is associated with resistances from past negative experiences connected to their sexual history—such as being disappointed every time they wanted orgasm but didn't get it, or forceful sex, or partners who used them.

I advised Ron: "Every time this happens to Cassandra, stop and release the pressure a little, take some deep breaths, and relax, but stay on the same spot until the pain moves. While you hold there, imagine yourself healing these past experiences by sending your love into the area. Then continue the stroking, perhaps connecting it with the Jewel Honoring so she associates the feelings with pleasure."

Since Cassandra was already very comfortable with Jewel Honoring, the G-spot–Clitoris Connection practice could work wonderfully for them. I encouraged Ron and Cassandra not to give up but to continue using the sacred-spot pleasuring as part of their lovemaking, even if only for five to ten minutes. I suggested it might take eight to ten sessions before the sensations of burning or urination actually turn into pleasure. When this happened they were to come and see us again. Some months later they told us they were ready for the next level, so we introduced them to multiple orgasms.

We continued to provide Ron and Cassandra with techniques that we knew would put them into a spin because challenges keep their sex life and their relationship alive and exciting.

11

Advanced Practices for Longer, Deeper Orgasms

Every man would like to know the secret to giving his woman the best orgasm she has ever had. In fact, you can't "give" a woman an orgasm— her orgasm belongs to her. What you can do is give her every possible chance of creating her orgasm with you.

Once your partner orgasms readily through Jewel Honoring you are ready to experiment with the sexual secrets in this chapter. The techniques are quite advanced and will work most successfully for a woman with whom you have been in a sexual relationship for quite some time, because you know her sexual responses well enough to do what is necessary at the right time and she has enough trust in you to let herself go to this level of orgasmic release.

Having the goal of achieving the longest and deepest orgasm ever can create a lot of performance pressure for both of you if you focus only on the goal. However, throughout this book I have talked about being in the present moment, stopping and enjoying what you are doing right now and not always focusing on the goal. When you are using these techniques remember to enjoy the journey, not just the destination. Reaching your goals can be fun if you have this attitude. The positive side of having sexual goals is that they can give you and your partner something to look forward to in the future so you won't become bored with your lovemaking. There is always more to explore.

As you try these advanced techniques be careful not to put pressure on yourself or your partner, or to give up and become disillusioned because it hasn't happened the way you thought it might. Remember: there are always challenges in life, always problems to work through. It's the same with your lovemaking. As you try these techniques for deeper and longer orgasms just think of it as part of your journey together into the extraordinary, and have fun with it.

DRAWING OUT THE ORGASM

As you are stroking the sacred spot, use your mouth on the jewel area at the same time. Continue this for a period of time until you start to feel the yoni muscles clenching. At this point try to simultaneously pull out the orgasm with your hand, matching your strokes with the contractions of the yoni.

Once you have mastered this technique, experiment with stopping use of your mouth just before your beloved is about to climax and, using only the hand that is already inside her yoni, start a beckoning motion, as if you are drawing the orgasm out. Focus your mind on an image or a feeling that you are psychically pulling the orgasm out of her. It's a great sexual secret to know how to do this.

Both these variations of this very powerful technique help your woman to have push-out contractions, rather than squeeze contractions, during her orgasm. Squeeze contractions are a kind of clenching action of the vaginal muscles and signify the first level of orgasm for a woman. A lot of men stop after the woman climaxes with squeeze contractions or immediately let go of their ejaculations as they try to come at the same time. However, there is another level of orgasm a woman can reach where she has a much fuller orgasmic release. This is accompanied by push-out contractions. Whereas squeeze contractions involve only the vaginal muscles, these push-out contractions involve contractions of the deep pelvic muscles as well as the vaginal muscles. When push-out contractions happen the woman feels that her cervix and uterus are pressing down into the yoni. This is where the term *push out* comes from. It's an amazing experience feeling this happening around your hand, let alone around your lingam.

These contractions usually only happen for a woman in a very high state of sexual arousal. It may take up to forty minutes of being in this state before she can experience this; sometimes only after many orgasms do push-out contractions happen.

ALTERNATING TECHNIQUE

Start with Jewel Honoring. If you are on your woman's right side, have the hood of the clitoris drawn back with the fingers of your left hand and stroke the clitoris and surrounding area with the middle and ring fingers of your right hand. When she is engorged and very close to orgasm, ask if you may enter her yoni. Take the middle and ring fingers of your right hand into the yoni, making sure they are well lubricated. Leave that hand steady and continue to stimulate her jewel area with the fingers of your left hand until you see her beginning to orgasm with squeeze contractions.

While she is having the squeeze contractions, start to stroke the sacred spot (G-spot) with the fingers of your right hand, at about the rate you were stroking her jewel when she climaxed. She may move straight into push-out contractions, but if she doesn't then continue to stroke the inside of her yoni, remembering to take one-second pauses between cycles. Keep doing this until you feel she has stopped getting pleasure and her energy is dropping. Now you can go back to the jewel, very lightly at first until she builds arousal again. Continue until she orgasms again with squeeze contractions, then switch back to the sacred-spot area once more. Continue this alternating until you create a full and deep orgasm with push-out contractions.

In chapter 10, when you were switching from the G-spot to the clitoris with the hands, the focus was on creating an association between the sacred spot and pleasure. The difference with the next technique is that the goal is to achieve deeper and longer orgasms.

Put several towels down for this practice because in heightened states of pleasure with G-spot stroking a woman may release vaginal fluids. As you practice this technique many times, your partner will experience a full orgasmic release with push-out contractions accompanied by an expulsion of female ejaculate, sometimes in large quantities. This is the amrita, the divine nectar discussed in chapter 9.

MULTIPLE ORGASMS

Many sex therapists say the difference between a single orgasm and a multiple orgasm is that, after single orgasm, there is a resolution phase during which sexual arousal and tension are significantly reduced. Multiple orgasms occur when a woman has a second, a third, or more orgasms without completely returning to that resolution phase.

Types of multiple orgasms include:

1. Compounded singles: Each orgasm is separated by a partial return to the resolution phase.
2. Sequential multiples: Orgasms two to ten minutes apart, with little arousal reduction in between.
3. Serial multiples: Sometimes these are experienced as one long orgasm separated by mere seconds or minutes, at most with no drop in arousal.

Whatever the type, all multiple orgasms are great. In 1953 Alfred Kinsey, the renowned American zoologist who conducted many surveys into human sexual behavior, declared that only 15 percent of women would ever experience multiple orgasms. From our studies Diane and I believe that any woman who is orgasmic can easily become multiorgasmic with the right man trained in sexual secrets. However, there are a couple of conditions that are necessary to ensure this. The first condition is that your woman understands her unlimited potential for orgasm, her unlimited shakti, and that the only reason she shuts down to pleasure after the first orgasm is that her mind shuts off.

The second condition is that you need to develop a way in which your woman reliably orgasms every time you make love. Maybe it's intercourse with her on top or maybe it's oral sex or perhaps it's with Jewel Honoring or with a vibrator. Whatever it is, don't use that technique for at least one week before doing the following practice. Save it for this session.

Let's suppose she always orgasms with oral sex, and so for this session that is the one you save. You might start the lovemaking with Jewel Honoring or whatever you like, but make it something that creates her first orgasm. Bring her to orgasm with something other than oral sex. Once she has orgasmed give her encouragement by saying something that will encourage her to go on. Immediately use oral sex to bring her to orgasm. When she comes this second time it may be a great breakthrough for her, and she will allow you to continue to pleasure her to another orgasm and another.

Once your partner has had the experience of more than one orgasm in a session, don't try to achieve this immediately again the next time you make love. It's my advice to leave it for a week or even a month before having another multiple orgasm session.

As your partner becomes more open to experiencing a multiorgasmic state, eventually you will notice the time between one orgasm and the next steadily decrease. Your beloved will be going from one orgasm to the next in only a few seconds. Eventually these multiple orgasms will merge into one long orgasmic experience that could last from several minutes to more than an hour.

SIMULTANEOUS VIBRATION

This technique is to be used once your woman is in a heightened state of sexual pleasure. Place a cushion under her sacrum or, ideally, take her into the cradle position. Cradle her in your arms with lots of pillows

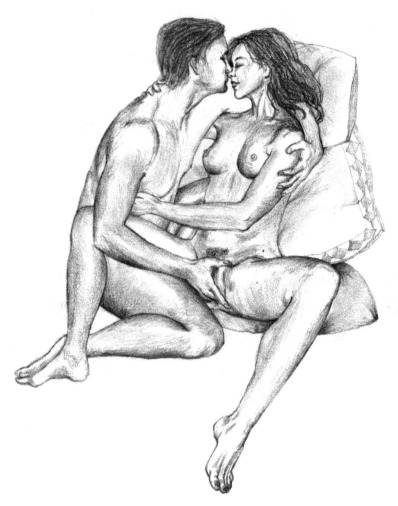

THE CRADLE POSITION

supporting you both. Have your ring and middle fingers of the right
hand on the sacred spot area and the palm of your hand curled around
so that the heel of the hand is touching the jewel area. Make sure to
have plenty of lubrication on your hand.

Start moving your hand so that you alternately stimulate the jewel
and the sacred spot. Once your partner is responding to this stimulation
start your hand vibrating, then stop and pause. Now use a slow-motion

movement from jewel to G-spot, G-spot to jewel, in and out, in and out, and then jewel and G-spot vibration again. You'll have to work out your own timing, tuning in to your woman's responses. Pause just at the point of orgasm, then slowly pull the orgasm out from the yoni or sweep the heel of the hand slowly and sensuously across the jewel area until the orgasm literally bursts out of her.

This is an advanced technique and is not for beginners.

A student told Diane and me: "There's nothing like it! Even the first time Andrew tried it with me I had such an intense orgasm my whole body was racked with spasms. The rapid vibrations with the palm of Andrew's hand just brushing over my clitoris were sending me crazy with excitement. Then he stopped with absolutely no movement and that's when the energy flooded my whole being and my body started to jerk. He repeated this several times and it was like I lost consciousness for a while, but then I remember when he started the slow-motion movement in and out of my yoni, from jewel to G-spot. And that put me into a new realm of pleasure. Then I could actually feel him pulling the orgasm out of me; there was an intense involuntary pushing from inside me, almost as though I was going to explode. Liquid literally gushed out of me. I felt totally relaxed and at peace for a long time afterward."

Andrew said: "I thought it was the sexiest thing I have ever experienced. I love being able to pull the orgasm out of Paulette. If I get the timing right, then as soon as I focus my mind I can see her respond. It's an unbelievable technique for us."

THREE ENERGY CENTERS

This is an extension of the previous technique. When you have your hand in this position and there is plenty of lubrication it's very easy to slip your little finger into the anus. This can be an area of intense sexual pleasure for many women, so you alternate between the three energy centers. Initially this may prove too much pleasure for most women to integrate. It may short-circuit her buildup of sexual energy; she may not be able to come like this. In fact, she could have difficulty afterward trying to release the amount of charge she has built up. However, with experience and more opening to her shakti and with you becoming more proficient at this technique, it may result in her best orgasm ever.

You can try a different combination of fingers in order to stimulate all three areas simultaneously. You can try two fingers on the G-spot, the little finger in the anus, and the thumb on the jewel. Sometimes you can hold this position with no movement so she gets to connect the energy produced from these three centers in her mind. Eventually she will get to a stage where she won't even be aware of what you are doing; she won't feel anything except her whole sexual center being opened with an enormous amount of energy.

In experimenting with all these techniques, make sure your hands and nails are clean and that the nails very short. Also, make sure you don't allow fingers that have been in the anus to slip into the vagina, as this can transfer bacteria from the anus into the sacred place, the yoni.

POINTS TO REMEMBER

- Remember to pause, stop sometimes, allow the energy to spread through the body. Go from fast to slow motion, to pausing and stopping often.
- Keep checking in. Touch your partner in intimate ways during the pleasuring.
- Open your eyes, speak, send her your love.
- Use plenty of lubrication.
- Don't put pressure on your partner or yourself to perform. Remember to have fun.
- Develop a loving, trusting relationship together so you can explore these things as teammates on a long journey into love.

CLIMAXING THROUGH INTERCOURSE ALONE

Statistics show that only about three in ten women orgasm from penetration only. Some women would prefer not to admit that they don't orgasm from intercourse alone. So the true statistics may be more like two in ten.

See if you can answer the following questions about the woman with who you are currently in a sexual relationship, or a woman with who you have been in a sexual relationship in the past.

1. Does she orgasm? How do you know? A lot of men don't know for certain because their woman may fake orgasm. Does your woman fake orgasm? Just because she makes sounds and moves as if she is climaxing doesn't mean she has had an orgasm. Have you actually seen her yoni during orgasm?
2. If she does orgasm is it rarely or sometimes or often? Almost every time or every time? With the knowledge and practice of sexual secrets for men and women there is no reason why it can't be almost every time. It's something you can work on as lovers and friends to achieve, not just as a goal but as part of your journey into love together.
3. Does she orgasm from self-stimulation?
4. Does she orgasm from your stimulation?
5. Does she orgasm on your lingam during intercourse?

In our seminars we have posed similar questions to help us determine at which level to direct our teaching. Couples are asked to respond anonymously, with each couple adding an agreed symbol to the top of their forms. No one, including us, knew who belonged to which symbol.

On matching the symbols, we consistently found that only 50 percent of the man's answers matched up with his woman's. We also found that in a typical group of twenty women, two or three never reached orgasm. Of the other seventeen, three could orgasm only through masturbation, eight could orgasm from his stimulation alone (usually through oral sex), and, significantly, only five could orgasm through intercourse alone.

We found that many couples had a routine where when the woman wanted to orgasm while her man was inside her, she would stimulate her jewel or he would stimulate her jewel with his hand until she orgasmed. It was surprising to find that only 25 percent of the women were able to climax solely from intercourse, without additional stimulation.

In this chapter I give you secrets that will assist your woman to orgasm on your lingam during intercourse. These secrets assume that she can orgasm through self-stimulation. If she can't then she might need to read some of the excellent literature available about becoming orgasmic, or she may want to work with a good sex therapist. It's easily solved in most cases these days.

HELPING YOUR PARTNER ORGASM DURING INTERCOURSE

Stage 1

This involves associating your lingam with her orgasms. You could use the method many couples use—that is, she learns to stimulate herself manually to orgasm while you are inside her. If you are on top of her, lean back and sit on your haunches so she can easily access her jewel. Otherwise get into other positions where it is easy for her to stimulate herself; her sitting on top of you or you entering from behind works well.

Another thing you can do to associate your lingam with her orgasm is to have her take your lingam in her hand and stimulate herself with the head of your lingam until she comes to orgasm, then slip your lingam inside her as she is coming. Another suggestion is get her so close to orgasm with other techniques that when you enter your partner it will only take a little stimulation to take her over the top. However, the problem with this is that when you change to the lingam from other techniques, her energy might drop and she can have trouble getting used to the new sensation. She may also get annoyed because as she was about to come you stopped, and it's as if you've taken it away from her because women love their orgasms. That could be dangerous! Whatever you try, the first stage of getting her to come on your lingam is to some way associate your lingam with her orgasms.

Stage 2

Continue practicing Jewel Honoring until your partner is totally at ease with you looking after her pleasure. It is a great break-through in a sexual relationship when a woman trusts you enough to let go, to surrender, to let you look after her orgasm. When she is masturbating she is in control. In Jewel Honoring she gives that control to you. That trust and surrender are very important to her being able to come on your lingam.

I can't overemphasize the importance of mastering Jewel Honoring. Once your woman comes regularly with you through Jewel Honoring you are well on your way to having her come on your lingam. It might take a year of practicing until you get to this stage, but the reward is worth it because there is nothing like your woman's pulsing, pumping yoni massaging and squeezing your lingam as she is coming all over you. It's not just technique with the lingam that will make her come. Something must occur in her mind about letting go of her orgasm to you, and that happens through Jewel Honoring.

Stage 3

The Jewel–G-spot connection is perfect to get the inside of the yoni connected with pleasure through the following sequence—Jewel-to-Pleasure, Jewel-to-G-spot, and finally G-spot-to-Pleasure.

You can use this same knowledge to connect the breasts with pleasure. Stimulate the nipples and jewel at the same time, then keep alternating. Eventually the nipples are connected with pleas-ure as much as the jewel. If you use this secret you can do it with the whole yoni—connect jewel to G-spot, jewel to back of yoni, jewel to inner-left side of yoni. You will need to make the same connection many times until the transmitters of pleasure to the brain connect up with that part of the body. Eventually the whole yoni can feel like the jewel.

This connecting process is very powerful. By connecting the clitoris with some other part of the body that particular part produces the pleasure itself. By developing the connection between the whole of the inside of the yoni with pleasure it is much easier for her to come directly on your lingam.

To make the association stronger, use the technique of stroking inside the yoni as she is coming, either through the sacred spot beckoning stroke or by moving your fingers in and out simulating the movement of the lingam, so that the inside of the yoni and orgasmic sensation become connected.

(Note: Vibrators can be great fun and extremely helpful to expand a woman's orgasmic potential. However, if you use them regularly eventually all of your woman's responses will be associated with the front of the yoni. The back of the yoni, deep inside where we often love to have our lingams, becomes less and less likely to give her an orgasmic response. All the energy is in the front of the yoni. Also, the electrical vibration isn't the same as human vibration, and she will have increasing difficulty coming during intercourse because it will be a different energy for her, one that is not associated with orgasm.)

Once you have mastered these three preliminary stages, your woman orgasming on your lingam is almost a certainty. Of course, once you move into this stage of her coming on your lingam it's imperative that you have great technique with your magic wand.

It's not the size of your lingam that counts, it's how you use it.

In most intercourse positions your lingam doesn't touch the jewel area, so unless you've developed stage 3 most likely the only way your partner can climax is if she is getting some stimulation on her jewel area.

Looking at the yoni it is obvious to see that if the lingam is stroking in and out of the vagina it is not going to touch the jewel. In most cases only your pelvis rubs against the jewel to stimulate it. So you need to find another position of making love where the lingam does stroke against the jewel.

Stage 4

The woman on top is sometimes the best way. However, if you are on top make sure you do a lot of stroking around the first third of the yoni before going in deeper. Get into a position where you lean over your partner so that your lingam is stroking the jewel area at the same time. It is easy once you know what you are trying to achieve, and if you have been Jewel Honoring a lot you are now as familiar with her responses as she is.

Only when your partner gets very excited do you enter with a couple of deep strokes. Keep alternating rubbing against the jewel with penetration of the yoni—deep into the yoni for a few times and then out again. Then vibrate or move your hips so your lingam is jiggling on the jewel area—get your whole body vibrating—then make several long, deep strokes. Repeat the jiggle again and then make deep circular rotating strokes. Move back out while jiggling on the jewel area again and then penetrate with deep strokes, alternating from one to another.

SETS OF NINES

The "Sets of Nines" is a famous Taoist technique; at this stage of your lovemaking you could try it or a variation of it. It goes like this.

Start with nine shallow strokes. This is in such a position that only the head of the lingam is allowed to enter the yoni—or preferably the lingam is rubbing up against the jewel area for nine shallow strokes. Then you go in for one long, slow, and deep stroke. Follow this with eight shallow strokes. Two deep strokes are then followed by seven shallow. Then three deep strokes are followed by six shallow. Each of these lovemaking "phrases" add up to nine, giving mathematics a whole new dimension!

Continue with four deep strokes followed by five shallow; then five deep, four shallow; six deep, three shallow; seven deep, two shallow; and eight deep, one shallow. Altogether there are nine sets of nine strokes.

Then you reverse the process, with nine deep strokes followed by one shallow stroke and eight deep strokes; two shallow and seven deep; three shallow and six deep. Continue subtracting deep strokes and adding shallow strokes until you reach a final set of one deep and eight shallow. This completes one cycle of nines, a total of 162 strokes. If you are highly skilled at lovemaking and have great control over your magic wand, you can try nine series of these phrases.

Of course you don't have to keep to this exact sequence. Do it in accordance with your partner's rhythms. You will feel when it is time to go in deep and when it seems time to come out shallow again. It's like playing music or dancing, with the shallow strokes rubbing against the clitoris and the deep strokes going deep into the yoni to the rhythm of your woman.

DRAWING OUT THE ORGASM
WITH YOUR LINGAM

As your lover approaches orgasm you may be inclined, as most men are, to thrust in more deeply to get your woman to come. Instead, try the opposite—concentrate on the out-stroke, not the in-stroke, and imagine that you are physically pulling the orgasm out. You have already learned how to do this with your hand if you have practiced the techniques in the previous chapter.

The challenge now becomes to do it with your lingam.

Remember, it is not only the number and kinds of strokes or length of the lingam, but the amount of love you transmit to your beloved through your lingam that makes all the difference between a good lover and an extraordinary lover.

Send your love and light to your beloved. Stop several times during your union and pour your love into your beloved through your lingam. See it as a transmitter of your heart energy of love and light.

12

It's Her Night

It's great to prepare a special night just for your partner, a night that makes her feel appreciated, loved, adored, and honored. Most women put romance high on the list of things they love best, so it is your challenge as an extraordinary lover on this special night to provide her with all the romance she could possibly hope for.

A lot of women complain that men are not romantic enough. Many men have been socialized to believe that it is totally not cool to be romantic with their woman, especially in front of their buddies. It is not part of being a real man. They don't need to "suck up" to their women; women are supposed to chase them.

I think this behavior toward women occurs for two reasons. First, the man may not know how to be romantic, and second, it's not part of his self-image. In fact, he probably feels silly being romantic.

If you feel a little silly being romantic it is time to work on changing that, because most women *love* romance.

It's my experience that men love romance too. They love romance once they take on the image of being a great lover. This is what I would like to encourage you to do on her special night. Be romantic, be extraordinary, think of romance as a way to transcend ordinary life, a means of transporting your beloved out of daily concerns—money, children, work, responsibilities—into wonderland, into a place where dreams come true.

"It's Her Night" is a title Diane and I use for a special night we include in our program when we take couples away on vacation seminars. I would like to give you some insights into what we do on these nights and hopefully these may inspire you to plan your own night with your beloved.

First of all we take people away from their normal daily life. We take groups on holiday together and pick a romantic place, because travel in itself is high romance. On this seminar we tell people this is a week where their lovemaking is their first priority; nothing else is more important. This has a powerful effect because in daily life it seems that everything else has become more important. People tell us:

- "My work is more important because we need money."
- "We have so many financial problems I can't think about sex tonight!"
- "My friends are more important!"
- "We haven't got time to make love, we must go to dinner tonight."
- "My sport is more important! I must ride my bike (play soccer, swim, or whatever) because that's my relaxation after a hard week's work!"
- "I just need to take my mind off things at night and watching television is easy!"
- "Sure the passion still comes up. We make love on Sunday morning or late at night after work, but it could be more often if we only had the time."

On our vacation week seminars, more time for lovemaking is what couples have. They have space, a break from routine and income-producing activities. It's a time for romance. Diane and I select a tropical island in Southeast Asia, the Italian alps, hot springs in Japan, or a palace in India.

For your romantic time together, your romantic night, choose a setting that is out of the ordinary, even if it is a motel not far from home. Wherever it is, choose a special place and spend a little more than you would normally. It may cost you three times your normal outlay, but how much is your night of romance worth? How much is your pleasure together worth?

Romantic dining is a key element. From our night in Italy I think of homemade pasta with Italian red wine and cheese. In Japan I think of sushi and hot saki. In Bali I think of fresh crab and tropical fruit salad. In India I think of tandoori chicken and a candlelit dinner in a palace on Lake Pichola. On your own night have something special to eat and drink together, preferably something you don't normally have at home or something that you have only on special occasions—caviar, French champagne, or any treats that excite your woman.

I will outline some of the things men have shared with me at our vacation seminars. "It's Her Night" usually takes place on the fifth night of the seminar.

On that day the men get together for a couple of hours and we share ideas on what we can do. Once everyone adopts the image of being great lovers they no longer feel embarrassed about doing romantic things. Then it becomes a lot of fun because they enjoy allowing the romantic within them to confidently emerge.

- Ron said he was going to fill the room with flowers and place petals on the floor for Valerie to walk on. He also intended to write words of love on cards all over the room, including on the mirrors.
- Peter said he was going to prepare a special bath for Kate, wash her all over, dry her, carry her to the bed, anoint her body with almond oil, and offer her special French perfume that he had bought her as a Christmas gift. Then he intended to give her a sensual massage to some romantic music.
- Kevin planned to borrow both Ron's and Peter's ideas and

then connect with his beloved in the yab-yum position while sending all his love to her heart and telling her how precious she is to him. Then he would ask her to allow him to serve her by honoring her jewel until she was fully engorged. Next he would ask her if he might kiss her yoni until she requested him to stop. He said he was going to take a box of chocolates with him and eat them one by one from her pleasure palace because oral sex was Helen's favorite form of lovemaking.

- Mark intended to arrange a selection of tropical fruits in a special basket from the resort restaurant, sit Lucy up in bed, put the tropical fruits next to her, and then dance and do a strip for her. As a joke, one of the men asked him to demonstrate. He agreed, provided some of us would do the same. He didn't actually do it for us but I suggest that you try it sometime to entertain your woman. Often in the world today we take our lovemaking too seriously, so making the night fun, entertaining, and enchanting for her is great.

- Tony suggested we could each sing a song for our woman. Most of the guys were too embarrassed to sing so Tony wrote down the words to a song for everyone. The song he suggested was "Can't Take My Eyes Off You." We each learned a few lines to say or to sing.

Some of the guys insisted there was no way they were going to sing, but they agreed to write a love letter to their woman. It amazed me how creative the men became. They got really excited about turning on a night to remember. The stories the next day were fantastic. Clearly they all had magical nights.

Lucy said that all her dreams of romance came true on the one night. She hadn't realized how creative Mark was and his dance was heaps of fun. In addition to a wonderful candlelit dinner followed by some great lovemaking, they had lots of laughs. Lucy said she wanted to bring more laughter into the bedroom when she got back home.

Prepare a night for your woman. Keep romance in your mind as you jot down some things you might include. Here is a list for you to choose from:

- candles
- flowers
- fruit
- wine
- bathe together
- music
- no phones
- no children
- fragrant oils
- foot massage
- whole-body massage
- dancing
- sing songs or create poetry
- make a dedication, a prayer for your lovemaking and your bonding
- breathe together connecting heart-to-heart
- energetic lovemaking
- Jewel Honoring
- worship her as a goddess
- generate compassion, love, and sexual ecstasy

Do whatever you feel will put your partner into a state of bliss. You will be surprised at the richness of your imagination as you create this night. As I said previously, many people believe that sex must be spontaneous, so they may initially resist planning "It's Her Night." However, it is my experience that you can prepare for sex and still allow the sexual experience to be free and spontaneous. In fact, there can often be more freedom within a structure than outside of one. Again, treat "It's Her Night" as just another thing you do in your range of lovemaking experiences together.

Most men like techniques, so preparing this night will be a lot of fun for you. Plan it step-by-step beforehand, but during the actual evening just do what comes to mind at the time. It's like training for surfing big waves. You prepare well and you know what to do, but when you catch a big wave it takes over and anything might happen. All the practice and preparation then pay off, but you don't think about that while you are on the wave.

You want a night to remember, so do it right. Make sure there is a rhythm to what you do that gradually builds throughout the evening. Good lovemaking can be like good music. Think of yourself as a composer of great lovemaking on "It's Her Night." Of course, within that composition the experiences are totally free. There are no limits to what might happen for your woman, for you, or for your relationship as a result. So prepare everything and ask your woman if you may look after her. Tell her it's her night to receive and you have prepared something very special for her.

The second approach to "It's Her Night" is for you to ask her, somewhere through the session, if she has any requests she would like fulfilled, whatever her fantasy may be. If she just says: "Make love to me" encourage her to be more specific, because women often have trouble asking for what they want sexually. You could reply: "I will for as long as you wish, but please tell me exactly what you would like me to start with. I would love you to ask me!" When she does, thank her and then do it. Tell her how much you enjoyed her asking you and encourage her to ask more often for what she wants.

The third approach is where your woman gets to request whatever she wants on the night and you honor all her requests. At our vacation seminars the women meet and Diane helps them break down any resistances they have to asking for what they want in bed. Each woman gets three requests for the night and everything is allowed. The women at first may feel self-conscious about asking for their wildest fantasies, but when they do the feedback from the men is that it is a real turn-on. The stories the next day are always a lot of fun.

After Tim had prepared the room for romance and Nola was in a comfortable and relaxed space, he asked her if she would like a tropical drink from the restaurant. She said she would, so he went off and ordered a couple of fantastic-looking cocktails, put them on a tray, and came back to the room. He decided before she came to the door that he would give her a special treat—he pulled his pants down and stood there naked with the cocktails in his hand. When the door opened, there before him was not his wife but another woman—in shock.

In his excitement Tim had knocked on the wrong door. Fortunately it was one of the women from our group, otherwise Tim might have been arrested. Of course, she was embarrassed, and so was he. He apologized profusely. It was very funny the next day during class when Tim and Nola shared this story with the group. Shelley, the unsuspecting "other woman," stood up and said: "Well it was interesting because when he came to the door I thought it might have been my present from my husband because he had gone away and said he was going to bring me back something special." It was certainly special, but it wasn't what she had expected.

By this stage in the seminar (day six) everyone feels very trusting of everyone else and many freely discuss the details of everything that happened the night before.

This is the way I would like love and sex to be for everyone, not a secret to be held but something to be freely accepted and talked about. Love and sex have the potential of giving us the greatest joys of being human. The great religions disagree on many things, but most agree on one thing: God is love. And that is good enough for me. In loving union I feel in touch with something greater than myself that makes my life worth living. I feel I get to touch of Heaven on Earth. One of my friends says, "We are just gods on holiday here on Earth." Making love is the best part of the holiday for me. What about you?

What I have shared with you in this book is very precious to Diane and me. You may be thinking to yourself: "This all sounds great, but I'll never be able to achieve it. I haven't even got someone I love right now." I want you to know that you have already started. By reading this book you've taken the first step on your journey to an extraordinary love life.

A lot of men have so much investment in their ego about already being a great lover that they will never take this step and, as a result, will never know the magic, the love, the joy, the ecstasy that is possible.

Once you put the secrets and techniques into practice your world changes; you'll find women will be attracted to you. And once you meet your beloved you will be able to touch her on every level of her being—physically, emotionally, and spiritually. To know a man, look at his partner.

What we all want is plenty of love in our lives. Love and sexual passion can continue to grow for you. Don't believe "experts" who tell you that it's unrealistic to expect to feel sexual passion with your partner after being together for a long time. That is not a reality for me or any man who does what it takes to develop artistry in sexual loving.

Thousands of people have already used these secrets to transform their love lives. I hope what we've shared with you in this book will open the door to your becoming a new breed of man—an extraordinary lover. May you bring joy to your woman's life and feel good about being a man.

For More Information

Kerry and Diane Riley teach seminars on ways of keeping love, intimacy, and passion growing in a loving relationship. Their workshop series "Tantra" is offered at three levels to suit individuals' and couples' needs. Consultations and other programs are similarly individualized.

Kerry and Diane hold four- to seven-day "Tantra Vacation Seminars" in Bali and Australia. These give couples the opportunity to combine a relaxing holiday with ecstatic lovemaking experiences, to encourage deep and heartfelt connections with one another, and to nurture their relationships on all levels—body, heart, and soul.

For women, Diane conducts the workshop series "Discovering the Tantric Goddess Within." In these workshops she facilitates reconciliation between the physical and spiritual aspects of female sexuality. Diane's book on women's sexual secrets is to be published next year.

For men, sacred sex sessions are available in Australia and the United States, with a modern day goddess of love introducing you to the arts of tantra for developing confidence and expertise in using the skills of sacred sex.

A correspondence course in tantric lovemaking, through tapes, CD, book, and videos, offers another way of furthering tantric lovemaking skills. Sessions include *An Exploration into Tantra, Ancient Arts for Modern Lovers, Sexual Secrets for Men,* and *The Body Sensual.*

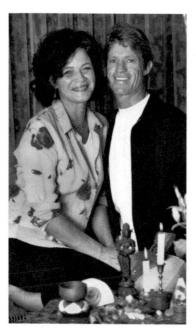

DIANE AND KERRY RILEY

The video *The Secrets of Sacred Sex—A Guide to Love and Intimacy,* co-created by Kerry and Diane with the video's producers, is a perfect accompaniment to this book. Beautifully filmed in exotic settings with visual but sensitive explicitness, six real-life couples demonstrate sacred sex methods adapted for Western lovers. The video provides a visual experience of many of the tantric practices outlined in this book.

For details on all programs and courses, and to order the videotape, see Kerry and Diane's web page: **www.tantragoddessoz.com.**

You can also contact Kerry and Diane at:

Spectra 2000 Pty Ltd.

PO Box 97

Avalon Beach, NSW, Australia 2107

(61)-2-9974 4724

Email: loveworks@ozemail.com.au

Bibliography

Anand, Margo. *The Art of Sexual Ecstasy*. Los Angeles: St Martin's Press, 1989.

Ashcroft-Nowicki, Dolores. *The Tree of Ecstasy*. London: Aquarian Press, 1991.

Baker, Jo-Anne. *Sex Tips—From Men Who Ride the Sexual Frontier*. London: Fusion Press, 2001.

Bethards, Betty. *Sex and Psychic Energy*. Novato, Calif.: Inner Light Foundation, 1977.

Brauer, Alan, M.D., and Donna. *ESO*. New York: Warner Books, 1983.

Britton, Bryce. *The Love Muscle*. New York: New American Library, 1982.

Brunker Stockham, Alice. *Karezza: Ethics of Marriage*. Moklumne Hill, Calif.: Health Research, 1983.

Chang, Jolan. *The Tao of Love and Sex*. New York: Dutton, 1987.

Chang, Dr. Stephen. *The Tao of Sexology*. San Francisco: Tao Publishing, 1986.

Chia, Mantak. *The Multi-Orgasmic Man*. New York: HarperCollins, 1996.

Collins, Larry. *Tantra: The Yoga of Sexual Bliss* (audiotape). San Francisco: Tantra Anima Productions, 1985.

De Angelis, Barbara. *How to Make Love all the Time*. New York: Macmillan, 1982.

Deida, David. *Intimate Communion*. (Deerfield Beach, Fla.: Health Communications, 1995.

Douglas, Nik, and Penny Slinger. *Sexual Secrets: The Alchemy of Ecstasy*. Rochester, Vt: Destiny Books, 1979, 2000.

Dumpleton, Harry. *Sex: A Four Letter Word?* Dee Why, Australia: Southwood Press, 1992.

Fisher, Helen. *The Sex Contract: The Evolution of Human Behaviour*. New York, Quill, 1983.

Frost, Gavin and Yvonne. *Tantric Yoga*. York Beach, Maine: Samuel Weiser, 1989.

Hayden, Naura. *How to Satisfy a Woman Every Time*. New York: Bible Publishing, 1982.

Hite, Shere. *The Hite Report*. New York: Macmillan, 1976.

Hooper, Anne. *The Art of Sensual Loving*. Victoria, Australia: William Heinemann Australia, 1992.

More University, Berkeley, California. Advanced Sexuality course.

Muir, Charles and Caroline. *Tantra: The Art of Conscious Loving*. San Francisco: Mercury House, 1989.

Mumford, John. *Ecstasy Through Tantra*. St. Paul, Minnesota: Llewellyn, 1988.

Neff, Dio Urmilla. "Tantra: A Tradition Unveiled," in *Yoga Journal,* April, 1983.

O'Connor, Dagmar. *How to Make Love to the Same Person for the Rest of Your Life*. London: Bantam Books, 1985.

Osho Times. *The Newspaper for a New Humanity*. Poona, India.

Rajneesh, Bhagwan Shree. *Tantra, Spirituality and Sex*. Rajneeshpuram, Ore.: Rajneesh Foundation, 1983.

Ramsdale, David and Ellen. *Sexual Energy Ecstasy*. Del Ray, Calif.: Peak Skill Publishing, 1991.

Von Urban, Dr. Rudolf. *Sex Perfection*. New York: Dial Press, 1949.

Stone, Hal and Sidra. *Embracing Each Other*. Novato, Calif.: Nataraj Publishing, 1989.

Welwood, John. *Challenge of the Heart*. Boston: Shambhala, 1985.

Index

Books of Related Interest

The Sexual Teachings of the Jade Dragon
TAOIST METHODS FOR MALE SEXUAL REVITALIZATION
by Hsi Lai

The Sexual Teachings of the White Tigress
SECRETS OF THE FEMALE TAOIST MASTERS
by Hsi Lai

Sexual Secrets: Twentieth Anniversary Edition
THE ALCHEMY OF ECSTASY
by Nik Douglas and Penny Slinger

Tantric Awakening
A WOMAN'S INITIATION INTO THE PATH OF ECSTASY
by Valerie Brooks

Celtic Sex Magic
FOR COUPLES, GROUPS, AND SOLITARY PRACTITIONERS
by Jon G. Hughes

The Yoni
SACRED SYMBOL OF FEMALE CREATIVE POWER
by Rufus C. Camphausen

The Phallus
SACRED SYMBOL OF MALE CREATIVE POWER
by Alain Daniélou

The Illustrated Kama Sutra - Ananga-Ranga -Perfumed Garden
Translated by Sir Richard Burton and F. F. Arbuthnot

Inner Traditions • Bear & Company
P.O. Box 388 • Rochester, VT 05767
1-800-246-8648
www.InnerTraditions.com

Or contact your local bookseller